*Complete Book of Beauty Treatments*

# Complete Book of Beauty Treatments

*Everything you need to know about
the latest products and methods*

## SANDRA SEDGBEER

Thorsons
*An Imprint of* HarperCollins*Publishers*

Thorsons
An Imprint of HarperCollins*Publishers*
77–85 Fulham Palace Road,
Hammersmith, London W6 8JB
1160 Battery Street,
San Francisco, California 94111–1213

Published by Thorsons 1994
1 3 5 7 9 10 8 6 4 2

A catalogue record for this book is available
from the British Library

ISBN 0 7225 2926 0

Printed in Great Britain by
Woolnough Bookbinding, Irthingborough, Northants.

# Contents

BELIEVING AS I DO that beauty has nothing to do with how you look on the outside, and everything to do with who and what you are 'inside', this book is dedicated to five of the most 'truly beautiful' women I know: my three lovely sisters, Marion, Mae and Pauline; my wonderful, irreplaceable 'mum', Vicky; and my very own flame-haired 'beauty', my daughter, Gemma.

'Though art much loved.'

# Acknowledgements

IN RESEARCHING and attempting to put together what I hope is a fairly comprehensive overview of the vast array of beauty treatments and products that are currently available today, I have had to rely on a large number of people for a great deal of information and help. Although it is not possible to acknowledge each and every one of them by name, I hope nonetheless that they are aware of the fact that they have my appreciation.

There are, however, a few people to whom I am especially obliged for their contributions to this work. I would particularly like to express my gratitude and appreciation to the following. To Bharti Vyas, a true pioneer of mind/body/spirit wellness, for providing me with some very useful sources of information; for the many patient hours she spent with me explaining the background to her own unique philosophies about 'beauty on the outside beginning on the inside'; and for arranging numerous demonstration treatments. My thanks also to Michelle Gardner of René Guinot for providing me with free access to her company's trainers, and for fearlessly arranging treatments without any guarantees that they would be rated favourably.

Thanks are also due, of course, to all the salon owners who wittingly – and unwittingly – provided both my own small team, and also scores of other testers, with the facility to experience a great many of the treatments detailed herein at first hand.

I am especially indebted to Roche Products Ltd., for providing me with vital research data on the use of vitamins in cosmetics, and for allowing me to plunder and plagiarise much of their own useful information on nutritional supplements for

Part 3 of this book.

I would also like to offer a very big thank you to two special ladies who have devoted a great deal of time, effort and energy to helping me research and organise the material for this book: to Anna Bowles, who spent hours poring over research papers, cuttings, brochures, and numerous scientific reports, and for setting up a sensible, practical and eminently workable filing system to house all my vital notes, transcripts, and literally hundreds of assorted sheets of data; and to my chief researcher, Sue Waterman, who heroically allowed me to subject her to innumerable therapies and treatments – most of which she found uncomfortable, unpleasant, and sometimes even unbearable, and only a few of which she actually enjoyed – for no reward other than a 'new pair of eyebrows'. Their efforts will long be appreciated and remembered.

And last, but by no means least, my thanks to Danial and Gemma for their patience and their forbearance in living for many months with a mother whose presence during the writing of this book was too often composed merely of the body, and not often enough of the mind and the spirit.

# Introduction

FOR AS LONG AS HISTORIANS have been recording world events, 'beauty' has played a major role in the affairs of humankind. Valued as highly as any priceless jewel, this ephemeral quality has, as history will attest, gained a reputation for inciting lust in the loins of men, and envy in the hearts of women of every culture, creed and race. Countries have waged war over it; individuals have been moved to commit murder because of it; and numerous family fortunes have been founded upon many a woman's desperate desire to possess it. Such is the power that societies have invested in beauty that the very word has long since ceased to be a description for something that is merely 'aesthetically pleasing to the eye', and become instead virtually a synonym for success.

Throughout history, different cultures have evolved their own individual definitions for beauty. This was, and largely still is, based upon whatever physical qualities were especially prized at the time. Although it is difficult to imagine – for those of us raised in a culture that esteems slenderness – that fat could ever be considered beautiful, many past societies have regarded fat people as highly desirable. In some parts of the world, such as Nigeria where fat is regarded as a symbol of wealth, this attitude still prevails today.

For as long as beauty has been valued as a priceless asset, women have been eager to experiment with a strange variety of peculiar ingredients and torturous treatments in order both to enhance or improve upon their natural looks, and to preserve the unlined features of their youth long past their middle age. Modern woman is no different from her early, primitive sisters in terms of her attitude to ageing. Both have the same dogged determination and spare-no-expense attitude to fighting age and the ravages that time brings to their faces and forms.

We may shudder with distaste at some of the more bizarre formulations that were used in earlier times. Roman women, for example, favoured a face paint blended from a mixture of minium (a red lead pigment still used in the manufacture of 'pink primer' paint), carmine and the excrement of crocodiles. In the 17th century, ladies risked blindness, paralysis and even death in order to make their eyes appear darker and more luminous by anointing them with belladonna juice, an extremely dangerous substance extracted from the poisonous plant deadly nightshade. One or two beauty treatments of earlier times have, however, been proven to work. Science has now established, for example, that Cleopatra's alleged insistence on bathing daily in asses' milk may indeed have had something to do with preserving the lady's legendary beauty. Fermented milk contains lactic acid, one of the naturally derived substances belonging to the group of compounds known as Alpha Hydroxy Acids (AHAs or 'fruit acids'). AHAs are currently being hailed as the most exciting anti-ageing cosmetic discovery to be made in years. It seems strange that, with all our technology, we are only now relearning and confirming what a long-dead Queen of Egypt accepted without question. I wonder how she knew?

Despite all the technological advances we have made, however, it is strange that a large majority of us still have not accepted one shatteringly simple truth. The secret of *true* timeless beauty will never be found in a tub, a pot, a jar or a tube. Neither can beauty be conferred on us by a few strokes of a skilled surgeon's knife. And though we tend to think of it as a marketable commodity, the essence of true beauty can never be manufactured, borrowed, bought or sold.

While it is true that every woman, regardless of her age or looks, believes she has a beauty problem that maybe, just maybe, one of the many treatments outlined in this book will solve, it is important to remember that even the most sublimely perfect woman (were such a creature to exist) would never be considered beautiful by everyone she met. Why? Because true beauty has nothing to do with youth, perfect bone structure, flawless skin, long slender legs, firm cellulite-free thighs, or a handspan waist. But beauty has *everything* to do with a person's inner qualities, such as genuine love of ourselves and of other people, energy, vitality, plus our enthusiasm for life and for all who share it with us. True beauty shines forth like a beacon from those who have attained perfect harmony between the physical, emotional, psychological and spiritual strands of their life. This means that every one of us is born with the potential to be as beautiful as we want to be.

This is not to suggest, however, that we should not be interested in looking after our physical bodies, or that it is wrong to take a certain amount of pride in the way we look, for these things are clearly important parts of the whole that makes each one of us unique. And if treating yourself to the occasional beauty treatment helps boost your self-esteem, then this, in turn, can only have a positive effect on every other area of your life.

It is also important to remember that we should not allow ourselves to become so caught up in our pursuit for physical perfection that we risk 'unbalancing' ourselves by focusing too much energy on too small an area of our 'self'. Likewise, we should not allow ourselves to become overly-influenced by the purely temporary dictates of fashion, or to become so preoccupied with our own body shape that we neglect to take sufficient care of the full range of our spiritual, emotional, mental and psychological needs.

For in the final analysis there is only one truth: regardless of what society may say to the contrary, true beauty cannot and should not be judged by what we look like. But it can and should be judged by *what we are.*

## The Beauty Industry

There is nothing intrinsically wrong with desiring to be attractive but, as with most human desires, the more we yearn for something, the more vulnerable we become. As the beauty industry exists only because of the natural insecurities that afflict us all, it has unfortunately attracted its fair share of charlatans throughout the ages. As long as we are prepared to spare no effort or expense in our pursuit of physical perfection, someone, somewhere, will always be keen to capitalise on our frailties by promising that they have the magic formula that alone can fulfil all our beauty dreams.

Today we have certain advantages when it comes to beauty treatments. Advanced technology enables scientists to subject new products to exhaustive testing procedures prior to their manufacture and widespread marketing. We also have a large number of regulatory bodies, industry watchdogs, laws, and official governmental regulations. These are designed specifically to protect the consumer from any unscrupulous companies or individuals whose only motive is to profit from our ignorance and/or our gullibility.

## The Aim of This Book

Beauty is an emotive subject. Our physical appearance has an enormous influence on our lives; indeed so much so that how we look often dictates how we feel, not only about ourselves, but also about the world around us and other people. Sadly, few of us pass through our formative years without gaining 'hang-ups' about our physical appearance. And even the lucky few who do manage to survive adolescence with wholly positive feelings about themselves are likely to be shaken by a degree of insecurity once time and gravity begin to exert their inevitable effect.

To be concerned with our looks is natural and understandable. Placing too much emphasis on a single aspect of our 'selves' can, however, become dangerous, for there is a very thin line between having a healthy interest in our appearance and vanity or self-obsession. And the closer we come to approaching that demarcation line, the more likely we are to lose our sense of perspective. This makes us vulnerable to the kind of hyperbole that feeds on our deepest dissatisfactions and insecurities. Unfortunately, this appears to be something that some factions of the beauty industry understand and utilise to expert – and highly profitable – effect. And while I am not suggesting that the intention is deliberately to mislead the public, the information accompanying most beauty products and treatments is undoubtedly selective. Not only does this make it difficult – and sometimes nigh on impossible – for the consumer to gain a true understanding of precisely what some forms of beauty treatments can and cannot achieve, but also to assess accurately whether or not a specific treatment is right for their own particular needs. It is for this reason that I have researched and written this book of beauty treatments.

Much as I would have loved to sample personally every single treatment covered in this book, the sheer quantity and variety of different products, therapies and treatments currently available is too vast for one person to investigate alone. It is fair to say, however, that virtually every salon-based treatment detailed herein *has* been subjected to a test, if not by me, then by either a member of my team of researchers and testers, or by independent testers whose reports (which have appeared elsewhere) have proved invaluable. What I have compiled is an overview of the respective merits and drawbacks of a vast array of treatments, which I hope is as unbiased as possible.

Once again, however, it is important to remember that experience is subjective – any treatment that may seem pleasant or effective to me may not necessarily elicit the same response in you. Conversely, it should be borne in mind that any treatment that may have been rated as ineffective by one tester could well prove to be successful with someone else. The comments that appear in this book can therefore be interpreted only as a collective *opinion*, and not as a definitive judgement, and any reader, or manufacturer, is perfectly at liberty to disagree with them.

To those of you who would like to try a particular treatment, but may be put off by my own or other testers' experience or opinion, the best advice I can offer is to say that, if you want it, and can afford it, go ahead and try it. For in the final analysis there is only one experience worth having, and that is your own.

If any specific treatments have been overlooked, this is either because they were not made known to me at the time of my research, or they were still too new to be widely available.

## Price-rating

The cost of the salon treatments covered in Part 1 of this book may vary quite considerably between countries, and even between locations in the same country. Whilst many manufacturers do provide salons with a suggested retail pricing structure, this is usually offered as a guideline only. When fixing their tariff of charges, salon owners will take into account a number of factors, including such items as the rental cost of their premises, insurance coverage, the cost of leasing, hiring, or buying equipment, and wages to their staff. Once these basic overheads have been covered, other factors such as the type of clientele they aim to attract, plus the relative income bracket of their potential customer-base will also figure in the equation. Thus, for example, a salon based in a prestigious location in the centre of a major city or capital will be more likely to attract a greater number of clients with a higher income than one located in the suburbs. Not surprisingly, therefore, this factor will be reflected in higher prices.

As this book is intended for international publication, and due to the variables outlined above, it would be difficult to quote the actual price a potential customer could expect to pay for any of the treatments covered herein. To circumvent this problem, I have devised a system of price bands. A symbol is given to each treatment which broadly equates to the average cost of the product or service. For example, where a treatment is priced low enough to be easily afforded by a housewife on a limited weekly household budget, this is denoted by the symbol ♉. As a further aid to the British market, I have also included an approximate equivalent in sterling based on the treatment being taken at a local, reasonably priced salon. A full description of the symbols is outlined below.

---

♙ 'Housewives' choice'. The cost of this treatment is unlikely to overstrain the weekly household account (up to £10).

♙ ♙ As affordable as a 'good cut and style' at a respected suburban hair salon (up to £25).

♙ ♙ ♙ The kind of price the average woman might reasonably be able to afford once every four to six weeks (up to £40).

♙ ♙ ♙ ♙ Not too much of a problem for female middle-management executives on a reasonably decent salary, middle-income housewives, and perhaps also those who believe beauty to be of far more value than eating for a week! (up to £75).

♙ ♙ ♙ ♙ ♙ Not to be indulged in too often unless you have access to a bottomless purse (up to £100).

♙ ♙ ♙ ♙ ♙ ♙ A rich woman's indulgence, or a terrific birthday gift, but enough to cause the average-income female to gulp if she were forced to foot the bill herself (up to £150).

♙ ♙ ♙ ♙ ♙ ♙ ♙ As above, only more so (up to £250).

♙ ♙ ♙ ♙ ♙ ♙ ♙ ♙ Only for those who regard spending what equates to the cost of seven to ten days in the sun as either 'a mere drop in the ocean' or good value for money (up to £350).

♙ ♙ ♙ ♙ ♙ ♙ ♙ ♙ ♙ A month's salary for many young working girls, or small change for the Ivana Trumps of this world (up to £450).

♙ ♙ ♙ ♙ ♙ ♙ ♙ ♙ ♙ ♙ Too high a price for the average woman to justify, unless the treatment is something she is determined to have at least once in her life, or one for which she is prepared to make sacrifices in order to pay for (up to £550).

♙ ♙ ♙ ♙ ♙ ♙ ♙ ♙ ♙ ♙ and above. These treatments are likely to represent either a year's savings and/or a once-in-a-lifetime experience for Ms Average Working Girl – unless she has a secret source of private income or a rich patron willing to foot the bill!

PART ONE

# Salon-based
# Beauty Therapy Treatments

# AROMATHERAPY MASSAGE

Aromatherapy is an ancient art that uses essential oils extracted from plants, bark, leaves, flowers, fruits, roots, seeds, spices and resins to treat a wide variety of ailments and disorders. Effects can be both physical and mental.

Although the ancient Greeks, Romans and Egyptians all believed in the therapeutic and healing properties of plant oils and essences, we owe much of our current scientific knowledge to the studies of René-Maurice Gattefossé (1881–1950). Although it was my intention originally to confine this section solely to beauty-salon treatments, further research revealed that there are a number of other therapies and treatments that are worthy of inclusion in this book. While some of these additional therapies may appear to have little association with a 'beauty treatment' in the accepted sense of the word, their physiological and psychological effects may, in turn, have a beneficial effect on one's overall physical appearance.

Although aromatherapy was used extensively throughout the Second World War to help heal wounds and scars, its present-day revival did not really begin until another Frenchman, Dr Jean Valnet, published a treatise on the subject in 1964. Today, essential oils are used in a number of different ways for their therapeutic effects. Some knowledgeable beauty therapists incorporate the use of essential oils in facial treatments to help a variety of skin problems and disorders, and more and more manufacturers are utilising plant oils in the formulation of many cosmetics to help promote healthy skin.

A fully qualified aromatherapist will have a knowledge of both anatomy and physiology. After taking a detailed medical case history and obtaining an overview of your general lifestyle, the therapist will prescribe and mix one or more oils together in a suitable carrier solution (this is vital as most oils should never be used 'neat' on the skin). The oil will then be rubbed into your body using massage techniques.

### Benefits and Claims

Because the oils are absorbed into the bloodstream via the skin, and also have an effect on the body's hormone-producing glands, it is said they can help relieve a surprisingly large variety of physical and mental ailments, from rheumatism and migraine to dermatitis and depression. It is also claimed that they can aid the body's lymphatic drainage process, thus helping to reduce cellulite and water-retention.

### Results

A personal favourite, aromatherapy massage is probably one of the most pleasant and deeply relaxing treatments that I have ever tried. Newcomers to this type of treatment should not be alarmed if they find that a treatment aimed at specifically stimulating detoxification of body tissues and lymphatic drainage results in a slight headache; this is merely a sign that the treatment is working.

Everyone I spoke to who had tried this treatment rated it very highly. Some claimed it had helped alleviate certain minor physical conditions; others said it had helped them cope more effectively with stress-related ailments.

### Value for Money?

As we now know that stress can be the starting-point for many of our modern-day ills, anything that can help promote relaxation naturally is definitely worth considering. An aromatherapy massage is beneficial on several levels: the massaging action helps break down fatty tissue, tone up flabby muscles and ease aching joints; while the therapeutic action of the oils helps alleviate symptoms of physical, mental and emotional origin. All in all, the benefits of this treatment make it well worth investing in on a weekly or fortnightly basis.

---

**AVERAGE PRICE**

ʊ ʊ

# AURICULAR THERAPY

Best described as a kind of 'acupressure of the ears', auricular therapy is a non-invasive, painless treatment. It involves the placing of a specially designed electrical implement, and sometimes magnets, on specific points of the ear relating to different organs and areas of the body. Electrical impulses are transmitted to the nerve endings in the ear via the implement.

## Benefits and Claims

According to Bharti Vyas, a highly respected London-based beauty practitioner, auricular therapy helps release blockages in energy flow from the brain, encourages the body's organs and systems to operate more efficiently, and also works on the external appearance of the skin from within. Auricular therapy may also be used to treat asthma, addictions such as alcoholism and smoking, arthritis, migraine attacks, digestive problems, and a variety of other disorders of nervous origin.

   In cases of persistent skin and beauty problems – such as acne, eczema and psoriasis, for instance – an on-going form of 'acupressure' treatment may be required between salon appointments. This involves attaching a small magnetic device to a point on or in the ear to which the client is advised to apply a small amount of pressure several times a day. Reports from testers indicate that this can create a marked improvement in certain skin conditions.

## Results

As with acupuncture, a session of auricular therapy may not create an immediate, noticeable difference in the way you look. Because of this, some people find it hard to judge its potential long-term benefits on the basis of just one treatment. After seeing the effects of several treatments on a male with an extremely severe case of acne, however, I can certainly attest to witnessing an almost miraculous transformation in both the appearance and condition of his complexion.

## Value for Money?

As this treatment is more popular, and therefore more widely available, in continental Europe than in most other countries, locating a practitioner within a reasonable distance from your home town may prove difficult. The additional cost of travel must be taken into account when assessing whether auricular therapy is the answer to your own particular beauty needs. For those who live in London, a treatment at Bharti Vyas's Paramedical Centre is excellent value for money.

# BEAUTY PADS

A relatively new innovation, Beauty Pads are a patented process invented by Professor Dr Romano Cali, a medical doctor and cosmetic surgeon. Beauty Pads are sterile cotton gauzes cut into anatomically correct shapes. They come coated in a variety of specific active ointment formulae for particular parts of the face or body.

Beauty Pads are adhered to areas of the body or face requiring treatment. As body temperature rises, the heat dissolves the natural vegetable substances contained within the ointment to allow their active ingredients to be released into the skin. Cali says that he developed the concept whilst using gauzes soaked in medicinal compounds for wounds and skin burns.

## Benefits and Claims

As no face has the same overall quality in terms of skin condition, texture and tone, Beauty Pads can be used to isolate and treat one specific area or defect, thus turning a normal facial into a combination treatment. The manufacturer's handbook, which appears to be a remarkably honest one, recommends the use of Beauty Pads in the treatment of the following problems:

- Face and neck wrinkles (except expression lines).
- Under-eye bags (caused by water-logged tissue, and not of

fatty origin).
- Oily unbalanced skin, including acne outbreaks.
- Sensitive, delicate, thin, dry, inflamed, sun-burned skin.
- Localised cellulite on the abdomen and hips.
- Firming – and in some cases lifting – of the breast, abdomen, inner thigh, face, neck and chin.

### Results

As I only discovered Beauty Pads shortly before completing this book, I was unable to put all the treatments to the test personally. However, after testing an under-eye pad at home, I noticed an immediate reduction in 'morning-after' puffiness, and a temporary disappearance of fine lines and wrinkles in the area covered. For best results, a course of six treatments at weekly intervals is recommended, with the client continuing treatment at home with a prescribed Beauty Pad cream.

### Value for Money?

If the results achieved on my home-test are anything to go by, this certainly appears to be a treatment worth splashing out on when you want to look your best, although I remain unconvinced as to whether a complete course could bring about a permanent result. Given that these treatments are not too overpriced, however, they are probably worth experimenting with as much as anything else that promises an equivalent result.

**AVERAGE PRICE**

Per Facial treatment – between 🌷 and 🌷🌷 depending on the salon, and whether a galvanic treatment is incorporated

Per Cosmetic Lifting treatment – between 🌷🌷 and 🌷🌷🌷

Per Body treatment 🌷🌷 Some salons offer reductions when booking a recommended course of 6 weekly treatments. As a guide, Beauty Pad creams for home use should generally cost around 🌷

## BLEACHING

Bleaching is an effective, albeit temporary, method of disguising superfluous facial and bodily hair. Bleaching works by lightening the hair until it blends in with your natural skin tone.

Although there are a number of over-the-counter products available for home use, if you are at all unsure about the DIY approach, it is advisable to put yourself in the hands of a qualified therapist. He or she will be experienced in both assessing and mixing precisely the right solution for your individual hair and skin type. Do be certain, however, to inform the therapist of any allergies you might have. If in doubt, ask for a free patch-test to be done beforehand. If no adverse effects are felt, it should be safe to continue with the full treatment a day or so later.

### Benefits and Claims

Bleach is effective in lightening hair on virtually any part of the body from your face – including the eyebrows, upper lip, chin, and downy areas such as the cheeks – to your arms and legs.

### Results

Bleaching is a fairly simple treatment that is usually satisfactorily completed in minimal time and with little fuss. Results can last up to four weeks before darker growth becomes visible on the face.

### Warning

Make-up should not be applied for at least 24 hours after bleaching facial hair. If treatment is carried out on your arms or legs, it is advisable to avoid hot baths, sun beds and all other forms of steam or heat treatment for a few hours afterwards.

| AVERAGE PRICE |
| :---: |
| ♙ |

### Value for Money?

For those who suffer from excessive facial hair, bleaching is a cheaper, less painful, and less time-consuming alternative to electrolysis. For larger areas of hair growth, such as on the arms, stomach, thighs and legs, bleaching is worth considering only as a last resort in cases where waxing, shaving and depilatory creams cause allergic reactions.

## BUST TREATMENTS

In France, where many of the world's favourite beauty treatments originate, no self-respecting beauty-conscious woman would consider any beauty regime complete if it neglected that all-important area between her neck and midriff. To the French, and many other continental women, omitting to pay attention to the bust and décolleté is tantamount to sacrilege.

Now, with the rest of the world having finally woken up to the French message that a woman's true age can always be ascertained by the condition of her cleavage, the bosom business is positively booming. Virtually every cosmetic house and beauty salon now offers one of a range of old and established, or newly-devised non-surgical treatments specifically aimed at softening, toning, and firming the décolleté, and lifting and improving the structure and contours of the bust.

## Decleor Bust-firming Treatment

After thoroughly cleansing the bust and décolleté of surface grime, the therapist will apply an exfoliating cream to the area to clear away any dry, dead skin cells. She will then massage the neck, shoulders and breast bone with essential oils containing lemon grass and rose, which are designed to stimulate and improve blood circulation and leave the skin feeling soft, tight and smooth. A poultice made of sesame seed, wheatgerm, plus tonic vitamins and minerals is then applied to nourish and replenish the skin, prior to a final cleansing and moisturising.

### Benefits and Claims

This treatment claims to help maintain the shape and firmness of the bust. It is said to be especially beneficial to those embarking on a slimming regime to help prevent any sagging or loss of firmness that often accompanies weight loss.

### Results

Difficult to assess, especially if treatment is taken whilst dieting. As this treatment is intended to *maintain* rather than *alter* the status quo, it is impossible to quantify whether the treatment was solely responsible for preventing any sagging or drooping of the breasts that might otherwise have occurred due to slimming.

### Value for Money?
As the price rating shows, this treatment hardly ranks as a 'housewives' choice'. This becomes all the more apparent when one considers that a course of three treatments is advised in order to achieve the best results (which could be translated as implying that 'one is not enough to make any real difference'); and that clients are also advised that, in order to continue the process, a special firming gel containing plant proteins, skin conditioners and moisturisers should be applied at home each night.

## Thalgo Bust-modelling Treatment

This treatment usually involves an hour-long session. Firstly, the area to be treated is thoroughly cleansed, then specially blended oils are massaged into the breasts, neck and shoulders. Next, a thick, heavy paste of firming marine extracts is applied over a layer of gauze and left to cover the breasts for 30 minutes. As the paste heats up it will dry to form a clay 'brassiere' which can be lifted off in one piece at the end of the session.

### Benefits and Claims
This is claimed to help firm, tone, tighten and lift the breasts.

### Results
An interesting, pleasant, relaxing and therapeutic treatment – but not necessarily an 'uplifting' one. As with many other bust treatments, the best results are most likely to be achieved after a course of treatment.

### Value for Money?
Debatable.

AVERAGE PRICE

ʊ ʊ ʊ

AVERAGE PRICE

ʊ ʊ ʊ

# CLARINS PARIS METHOD TREATMENTS

Created by Jacques Courtin-Clarins, founder of the famous cosmetic house which bears his name, the Clarins Paris Method range of treatments are all said to be based on a 'totally unique massage technique' that has been shown to be 'outstandingly effective in improving the body's blood circulation and lymph draining systems'. A former medical student turned physio-therapist, Clarins decided to diversify into the field of beauty therapy after enthusiastic claims from his female patients that his technique was responsible for not only improving their medical conditions, but also for the effects it appeared to have on their skin.

A cornerstone of the Clarins' philosophy is the assertion that the only tool a beauty therapist requires is her hands. According to Clarins, the trained hand has unrivalled flexibility of move-ment, position and pressure, which not only makes it much more effective than a piece of equipment, but also ensures that a treatment never dates.

Moreover, according to his company's publicity machine, Monsieur Clarins asserts such strict control over the training and practice of his technique, that there are only 15 training managers in the world who own the rare privilege of having been personally trained by him, all of whom are required to retrain with him in Paris at least every six months. Each of these training managers is said to train in turn only a select number of beauty therapists who, at the commencement of training, are required to sign a contract stating they will never divulge the secrets of the Paris Method to anyone. And even then, trainees are not deemed worthy of being a qualified Clarins therapist until they have attained the highest standard of technique by passing a final examination. Sounds like tough going.

Although I am personally wary of any treatment that is surrounded by so much secrecy, mystery and what sounds to me suspiciously like hyperbole (well, what else can you call it when they describe this as the 'Rolls Royce' of their own treat-ment range?), there is no doubt that both the Clarins Paris

Method Facial and Body treatments are enormously popular worldwide.

The range of different treatments available are now listed. Please note that most sessions last for one hour, and all treatments are preceded by a 15-minute consultation.

## Paris Method Body Treatment

This is designed to actively stimulate the circulatory and lymph-drainage systems to help eliminate puffiness and 'uneven spongy skin texture,* that is most commonly found on the buttocks, thighs and upper arms.

## Paris Method Bust Treatment

Similar techniques to those described above are used in a treatment of the same duration to help improve the condition of the skin and the shape of the bust.

## Facial Treatment

This treatment commences with a thorough cleansing of the face and neck, followed by a lengthy massage incorporating the use of specific Clarins products designed to stimulate intensively circulation and lymphatic drainage. It is claimed that this treatment is especially effective in treating puffiness, dull skin tone and broken capillaries.

## Firming Bust and Neck Treatment

This incorporates the massage technique with specialised intensive bust-firming products.

---

*Considering that France is one of the few countries in which cellulite is not only taken seriously, but also is regarded as a medical condition, it seems rather odd that Clarins a – French organisation and proud of it – should be so coy about using the term cellulite.

## Prescription Facial

A facial tailored to treat specific problems such as sensitivity, dryness, congestion of the skin, fine lines and loss of firmness.

## Purifying Facial and Back Treatment

This is specifically aimed at treating young or problem skin that is prone to break-outs.

## Relaxing Body Treatment

Described as the perfect antidote to a stressful life, this massage concentrates on the back, legs, stomach and arms using a special formulation of 100-per-cent pure plant oils known for their relaxing and restorative properties.

## Relaxing Facial

A treatment specifically aimed at both men and women with stressful lifestyles. The first 20 minutes is devoted to deep cleansing of the face and neck. This is followed by 40 minutes of relaxing, tension-easing massage starting with the face and moving on to the back and shoulders.

## Top-To-Toe Refining Treatment

A combined treatment for face and body, commencing with exfoliation of dead surface skin cells to deep-cleanse, smoothen, soften and brighten the skin, followed by a soft-ening and relaxing top-to-toe massage using own-brand pure plant face and body oils.

### Benefits and Claims

All Paris Method treatments are said to incorporate a com-plicated series of over 70 massage movements which take place in a specified order. Each treatment also involves the application of specialised plant-based products tailored to individual and specific concerns. All treatments are preceded by a 15-minute consultation.

### Results

Like many other face and body treatments that incorporate massage, the Paris Method range undoubtedly has the therapeutic benefit of easing away tension and leaving you tremendously relaxed. As to how well they actually live up to the remedial benefits implicit in their promotional 'blurbs' is virtually impossible to assess after just one treatment.

The bust treatment has received favourable reports from several independent testers who claim to have seen a marked improvement in the tone of their busts after combining one or more salon treatments with self-massage for three-months.

### Value for Money?

If you are into massage in a big way, and you lead a fairly stressful lifestyle, it might be worth investing in a regular Paris Method Top-To-Toe Refining Treatment as there is no doubt that this can have considerable physical, psychological and emotional benefits. The bust treatment requires purchasing the appropriate Clarins products which will increase the overall cost of treatment.

The key deciding factor in terms of value for money must surely rest on your level of disposable income. As Clarins have attracted their fair share of aficionados among the wealthier set, we must assume that, at least as far as these women are concerned, regular facial sessions are worthwhile. With regard to the less well-off, however, my own view is that, while a facial treatment would make a welcome gift, they are too pricey to be anything other than an occasional treat. If it meant having to go without something else in order to save up for a monthly Paris Facial, I would rather save up for a few extra months and spend my money on another form of treatment that would ensure a more tangible result.

---

**AVERAGE PRICE**

Approximately

**ᴈ ᴈ**

for most 1¼ hour
treatments

*Best-value Treatment in the Range*
Top-To-Toe Refining Treatment.

## CELLULITE TREATMENTS

According to most members of the medical profession, cellulite
– which affects almost 80 per cent of women – is a myth.
Strange, then, that what is regarded as a 'non-existent'
condition should be able to support a multi-million pound
industry in which virtually every major cosmetic and publishing house now has a finger. Stranger still that there should
now be a plethora of specialised clinics springing up all over
the western world whose only *raison d'être* is the treatment
and ultimate elimination of cellulite.

Regardless of what the orthodox medical establishment has
to say on the subject, and despite the fact that the word itself
does not appear in any medical textbook or dictionary, not
only does cellulite exist, but its stubborn presence is also a
constant source of misery, not to mention intense embarrassment, for millions of women throughout the world.

By now it is common knowledge that you do not have to
be fat to have cellulite. In fact, you do not even need to overeat
to suffer from it, although *what* you eat could be a contributory factor, as certain foods can exacerbate the problem.
Interestingly enough, however, the ugly, bumpy bulges and
dimpled 'orange-peel' skin that characterises cellulite only ever
seem to affect women – not men. While there are, as yet, no
proper medical studies on the subject, the most likely explanation is that cellulite is linked to the female hormone
oestrogen. According to many specialist health writers, including health expert and author, Leslie Kenton, and medical
journalist, Liz Hodgkinson, both of whom have investigated
the subject in depth, cellulite seems to be caused by a combination of poor circulation, a sluggish lymphatic system, and
the presence of oestrogen in the body. In fact, research suggests
that the higher the level of oestrogen in a woman's body, the

more likely she is to develop cellulite. Some 'experts' believe that taking the contraceptive pill can increase the likelihood of cellulite developing for some women.

Research has shown that cellulite is not the same as ordinary fat. It is formed when poorly regulated blood flow within the tiny capillaries serving the fat cells causes plasma and excess fluid to seep into the spaces between the cells. In time, thickened fibrils of collagen surround the cells forming lumpy structures known as micronodules. Wastes accumulate, nutrients vital to the cells' healthy growth become blocked, and fluid and toxins become trapped in the tissue, unable to escape in the normal way via the lymphatic drainage system. Women most at risk are those with sedentary lifestyles who consume an above-average amount of junk food (or other foods containing high levels of additives, flavourings, and preservatives), alcohol, caffeine and tobacco.

As mentioned earlier, there are countless products, potions, programmes, lotions and creams currently being advertised as the 'answer' to every cellulite-ridden woman's prayers. But as it is not within the scope of this book to cover over-the-counter products and preparations intended to be used at home, I shall offer no further opinion on these other than to say that, regardless of its constituents, no single product will shift cellulite permanently on its own.

Not surprisingly, as lifestyle factors are the major contributory cause of cellulite, the only reliable method of effecting a permanent cure seems to involve those programmes that address *all* these factors, and not just one or two of them. This has been taken into account in my review of the anti-cellulite treatments listed below.

## The Cellulite Clinic

This specialised clinic, based at the London College of Massage, is distinctive for two reasons: not only was it the first clinic to be established in Britain specifically to help women deal with the problem of cellulite, but it also happens to be the first to base its entire programme on a totally holistic approach.

The three-month programme (Option 1) commences with an initial hour-long consultation with a qualified nutritionist in order to establish the dietary, nutritional, health, stress and lifestyle factors that may be contributing to your cellulite problem. Any necessary dietary alterations will then be advised. The emphasis is on aiding the detoxification process and the release of cellulite deposits, and building optimum health and vitality. Nutritional supplements may also be recommended. This is followed by a detailed explanation of the benefits and a demonstration of the techniques of dry-skin brushing to improve circulation of the blood and lymph and speed up the elimination of toxins stored as cellulite.

Then comes the embarrassing part – a detailed assessment of your body. All the areas where cellulite exists are noted on a chart which will be used to monitor your progress. After that, you can relax and enjoy 90 minutes of relative bliss, while your own highly qualified personal masseur treats your entire body to a deep massage session, with special devotion to your cellulite zones. You will be taught a number of specific massage techniques to carry out daily at home, using specially selected aromatherapy oils, to help speed up the elimination of cellulite deposits.

The next step involves devising a three-month programme that is individually tailored to suit your needs. This will include a monthly consultation with your nutritional therapist, and a one-hour massage at the clinic one to three times a week. Throughout the programme your progress will be closely monitored by your own therapist, who will also advise you of any adjustments that may need to be made.

For those who would find it too difficult to visit the clinic each week for their treatment, a further option is available (Option 2). This special package comprises an initial visit, incorporating everything outlined above from the nutritional consultation right through to the massage treatment and self-massage advice session. It also includes a basic nutritional pack, dietary advice sheets, skin brush, aromatherapy oils and a copy of a book entitled *The Massage Manual*, written by Fiona Harrold, Director of The London College of Massage (published by Headline in Britain and Sterling in the United States).

### Benefits and Claims
No instant miracle claims are made for this treatment. Instead, the Clinic takes a refreshingly truthful stance in acknowledging that there are no overnight cures for cellulite. It sensibly stresses that the only way this problem (which, in many cases will have taken months, and perhaps even years to accumulate) can be treated successfully is through a concentrated, long-term, holistic approach that encompasses every area of your lifestyle.

### Results
The results of this programme are directly related to the level of commitment shown by the client. Those who have followed the programme to the letter have been very successful in eliminating their cellulite problems.

### Value for Money?
There is no doubt that, to a degree, this programme is effective, but the price of the full three-month treatment, if not a deterrent, could certainly be a huge obstacle for many women. For those who can afford it, however, the crucial factor in assessing whether this treatment represents good value for money lies not so much in the amount of money it costs, as in the amount of effort each client puts into the programme. If you are not prepared to invest the necessary time and effort in skin-brushing and self-massage, to make some radical changes in your diet and lifestyle, and to commit yourself wholeheartedly to every single part of the programme, then regardless of how much or how little cash you have, you would be ill-advised to invest any of your money in this.

Conversely, if your cellulite bothers you so much that you are prepared to do whatever it takes to get rid of it, and you

---

**AVERAGE PRICE**

Initial nutritional consultation
ꟓ ꟓ ꟓ

Initial massage treatment
(90 minutes)
ꟓ ꟓ ꟓ

Follow-up nutritional consultations
(30 minutes) ꟓ ꟓ

Massage treatments
(one hr) ꟓ ꟓ ꟓ

Dry-skin brush
ꟓ

Nutritional supplements (30-day supply) – from ꟓ ꟓ

Cellulite Massage Oil (100 ml) – from
ꟓ

Cellulite Bath Oil – from ꟓ

Estimated total cost of a three month programme based on one treatment per week ꟓ ꟓ ꟓ
ꟓ ꟓ ꟓ ꟓ ꟓ ꟓ

Option 2
ꟓ ꟓ ꟓ ꟓ ꟓ ꟓ

are 100-per-cent certain that you will not allow any of your old bad habits to sneak back into your lifestyle to sabotage your success at a later date, then this could ultimately prove to have been worth every penny of its price.

If you are tempted to choose Option 2 on the grounds that you will get the same information and guidance offered to Option 1 clients at a fraction of the cost, think again. Can you really be certain that you have enough will power to get through the programme on your own? Cutting corners price-wise will be a false economy if the effort of going it alone (without the benefit of weekly massages and consultations to help reinforce your determination) proves so great that you abandon the programme half-way through.

## Cellulolipolysis

A relatively new technique, cellulolipolysis is, as yet, only available under medical supervision. Promoted as 'pain-free transcutaneous electrotherapy', this treatment is not unlike acupuncture in that it involves having a number of very long thin needles inserted into your body. These are wired up to electrodes which deliver an irregular pulse into the fatty tissue to stimulate a number of functions. Although it sounds pretty horrifying, and looks even worse, I am assured that it is not at all uncomfortable.

At an initial consultation, your suitability for treatment is assessed, and your basic medical requirements are noted. This includes: recording your medical history to establish any possible contra-indications; blood, urine and nutritional analyses; an assessment of your metabolic and hydro-sodium equilibrium to identify your sodium/potassium balance.

A course of treatment consists of six one-hour weekly sessions. At each visit, a number of fine, sterile needles connected to electrodes are inserted between 3–5 mm deep into the subcutaneous fatty tissue where cellulite exists in your body. A 9-volt current is then passed through the needles at irregular intervals in order to raise the body temperature, improve local blood micro-circulation of the poorly drained cellulite areas, and increase cellular activity. This is claimed to activate the fat cells to release excess water and waste fat. Dietary changes are recommended to assist the process, as is a programme of exercise designed to help boost your metabolism.

### Benefits and Claims
A local improvement of the skin texture, the elimination of, or an improvement in, the dimpled, orange-peel effect of cellulite, and a reduction in girth equivalent to between one and two dress sizes.

### Results
According to the Association of Aesthetic Medicine, 'over 50,000 people have been successfully treated in several European countries where negative results were recorded in less than two per cent of cases'. Moreover, they also claim that medical trials conducted by the nuclear physics department of one of London's leading teaching hospitals proved conclusively that treatment is successful in 85 per cent of cases, with the remaining 15 per cent showing 'a significant improvement'. Results are said to last for at least four years, which, to date, is the maximum period during which trials have so far been conducted.

### Value for Money?

**AVERAGE PRICE**

Six week course
👜👜👜👜👜👜👜
👜👜👜👜

If you are seriously contemplating liposuction, then this has to be a better-value alternative for your money – if only for the fact that it is cheaper (just!), non-invasive, non-disruptive to your life, and leaves no scars. In any other circumstance, however, I would be inclined to give it a 'doubtful' rating, as far as value for money is concerned.

## Decleor Anti-cellulite Treatment

After an examination to assess the type of cellulite you have

– such as whether it is hard or soft – and how difficult or easy it will be to treat, the therapist will recommend the number of treatments you should have, and offer a healthy diet and exercise plan. Each treatment session consists of exfoliation, massage, and application of both a warm treatment mask and a thermal gel.

## Benefits and Claims
Decleor claim good results can be achieved providing the client pays rigorous attention to the diet and exercise plan.

## Results
The only truly uncomfortable part of this treatment is the massage – but as cellulite tissue is more painful under pressure than normal fat, any form of massage in this area is likely to hurt a little. After a course of treatment your skin should definitely feel much softer and smoother, but it will not make much of a dent in the appearance of your cellulite unless you are also prepared to put in a lot of personal effort away from the salon.

## Value for Money?
I would give this a 'so-so' rating. On the one hand it could be considered a good 'kick-start' treatment to reinforce your motivation at the beginning of a diet or anti-cellulite programme. If you are really dedicated to banishing your cellulite, however, the same results could probably be achieved just as easily – and a lot more cheaply – by combining regular self-massage and skin-brushing sessions with a sensible detoxification diet and exercise regime.

| AVERAGE PRICE |
| :---: |
| Single treatment – a fraction over |
| 𝗨 𝗨 |
| Course of six sessions – a fraction under |
| 𝗨 𝗨 𝗨 𝗨 𝗨 𝗨 |

## Ionithermie Anti-cellulite Treatment

Ionithermie treatment for quick – albeit temporary – inch loss has been around for a long time. Now that cellulite has become 'big', the manufacturer has refined both the programme and technique of treatment to encompass this aspect.

After taking your measurements and assessing the areas to be treated, the therapist will massage you from waist to knee using ampoules of 'slimming' gels containing plant and seaweed extracts claimed to promote detoxification. Once this has been completed, she will attach a set of electrode pads to the problem areas. A layer of quick-setting thermal clay will then be applied, the machine will be switched on and for the next 30 minutes a series of rhythmic electrical impulses will set your muscles contracting and relaxing.

## Benefits and Claims

The faradic current is said to stimulate circulation to help break down fatty deposits, release fluids trapped between the fat cells, and also to stimulate lymphatic drainage. The presence of the thermal clay helps to promote sweating which is one of the body's key waste-disposal methods.

## Results

As you might expect, treatments result in softer-feeling skin, a slight smoothing out of bulges, and an immediate, but usually temporary, inch loss around hips, bottom and thighs. The inch loss appears to be brought about by the compression and detoxification involved, which temporarily forces trapped water out of the tissues. Although this can be an ideal treatment if you want to look good in a favourite outfit on a special occasion, one session alone is not likely to be enough to result in either a permanent inch loss or a noticeable reduction in cellulite. A course of five treatments in conjunction with a detoxifying diet and exercise regime might help prolong the effect, but unless you are prepared to commit yourself totally to a healthier way of living, it is unlikely you will be able to maintain your new look for very long.

## Value for Money?

From a slimming standpoint, if you are prepared to pay a high price for a drastic and very temporary inch loss, it might just be worth shelling out on one treatment. If shifting cellulite is

---

**AVERAGE PRICE**

Single treatment
ṹ ṹ ṹ ṹ

Course of five
treatments
ṹ ṹ ṹ ṹ ṹ ṹ ṹ

Most salons recommend that a course of five treatments should be taken over 10–14 days. Some salons may offer special packages incorporating either one free salon treatment, or a free home-treatment pack of massage gel when you book a course.

your prime objective, five sessions might get you nearer to your goal, but you would be well-advised to weigh up the pros and cons first. After all, you would have to be either fairly cavalier with your money, or reasonably certain that you could commit to a permanent change in your lifestyle to invest a sum of this kind in something that could so easily fail to provide any real lasting benefit.

## A Final Word on Cellulite Treatments

Overall, it is difficult to enthuse about any one single technique, type or brand of cellulite treatment that is currently available, as all rely a great deal on the client's own commitment and effort for their results. Thus, if you are truly determined to banish cellulite from your life, committing yourself to a regular programme of daily skin-brushing, and self-massage, and combining this with a sensible detoxifying diet is just as likely to achieve a result comparable to any of those promised by specialist cellulite clinics and salons – without the cost. And if you cannot commit to such a regime on your own, then it is highly unlikely that the mere fact of paying for treatment will sustain your determination throughout the duration of a course that may last for several weeks.

My advice to the money-conscious is: test your will power first. If you are unable to tolerate the necessary changes to your lifestyle for as long as it takes to witness a result from your own daily efforts, you might as well save your money, and save yourself disappointment too.

# CHINESE HERBALISM

Not to be confused with a beauty treatment, Chinese herbalism is nonetheless a proven method of treating a number of potentially disfiguring skin problems, including eczema, psoriasis, dermatitis, acne-rosacea and urticaria.

Traditional Chinese Medicine (TCM) has been used successfully to alleviate and treat a number of ailments for more than 3,000 years. Based on the premise that most skin conditions (as well as many chronic maladies) reflect an imbalance within the body, TCM aims to look beyond the presenting condition in order to evaluate the *cause* and to treat the underlying deficiencies or excesses in the system.

Medicines prescribed by a Chinese herbalist are tailor-made to treat both the individual and the condition. After an initial consultation lasting around one hour, the practitioner will make up a prescription to be taken daily over the next 7–14 days. This will consist of a combination of up to 15 (out of a total of 120) different herbs. In some cases these may be offered in tablet form, but it is more usual for them to be given as a package of mixed herbs to be taken home and boiled and drunk as a decoction, or tea.

Although some patients are at first put off by the taste and appearance of the 'tea' (which many describe as a foul-tasting brew), the fact that this is often a last resort is sufficient incentive to make them 'grin and bear it'. For those with a real aversion to strange tastes, such as children, the brew can be made a little more palatable. Certain clinics, such as the Chi Clinic in London, find that the best approach with children is to remove the mystery – and any initial resistance to drinking the tea – by simply allowing them free access to the Clinic's pharmacy where they are encouraged to wander around touching, smelling, and asking questions about the herbs.

Treatment usually takes between four and six months, depending on the severity of the condition. Patients start by taking a more concentrated form of medicine which is gradually reduced as their condition stabilises. Some patients are also encouraged to continue with the use of any topical creams or preparations prescribed by their own doctor or skin specialist that may be helping to alleviate their immediate symptoms, but this is gradually scaled down, and ultimately dispensed with, once the TCM treatment begins to take effect.

## Benefits and Claims

Ruth Delman of the CHi Centre in London says that traditional Chinese herbalists never use the word 'cure' as they 'do not believe it is possible to cure a weakness in the system, only to rectify it or alleviate it for a longer rather than a shorter period'. TCM is said to be particularly beneficial in treating and alleviating a variety of skin conditions, including eczema, psoriasis, urticaria, dermatitis and acne rosacea.

## Results

Despite the fact that no guarantees are offered by the practitioner, TCM is nevertheless credited with effecting a number of near-miraculous 'cures' by hordes of grateful former sufferers of eczema and psoriasis. Trials conducted at the Great Ormond Street Hospital in London on a number of children suffering with eczema revealed a 60 per cent improvement in 60 per cent of those treated with TCM.

## Value for Money

Excellent. Having known several people who have been moved to try TCM purely as a last resort, and having been impressed by the results I have personally witnessed, I would have no hesitation in recommending this form of treatment to anyone suffering from eczema or psoriasis.

**AVERAGE PRICE**

Initial one-hour consultation plus seven bags of 'brew' (enough for one to two weeks) ♨♨♨♨

Follow-up consultations – free
Additional bags of 'brew' ♨♨♨

# COSMETIC CAMOUFLAGE

Having a disfiguring skin condition can create enormous emotional, psychological and social pressures on a person. Apart from the ever-present self-consciousness factor, normal social encounters that others take for granted can all too often be turned into an ordeal for anyone whose appearance differs from the norm. Although people do not generally mean to be unkind, they little realise how their curious stares or deliberately averted eyes can reinforce a feeling of hopelessness, inadequacy or rejection in someone whose appearance is visibly marred by scars, blemishes, birth marks, port wine stains, vitiligo, or some other unfortunate physical imperfection.

Whilst recent innovations in medical science, surgery and laser technology are offering new hope to many people afflicted with facial disfigurements, certain conditions still remain for which there is either no known, or at best only a partial, cure. For sufferers, cosmetic camouflage represents the only hope they may ever have of disguising or diminishing the appearance of those facial flaws.

Pioneered by the Red Cross, and available through their Community Programme, training in cosmetic camouflage techniques is available free, but only on referral by a doctor, to anyone who would benefit from this service. Specially trained Beauty Care therapists, working on a voluntary basis, advise clients on how to achieve a good skin-colour match, and teach them, step-by-step, how to apply the camouflage creams to their skin and set them. As all the camouflage creams contain over 38 per cent pigment, they are much denser and therefore far more effective than ordinary foundation creams which are only 7 per cent pigment-based. Moreover, because they both contain a sunscreen and also are waterproof, they will remain effective even when swimming or sunbathing. Sessions continue until clients have gained sufficient experience and confidence to enable them to perform the process unaided.

In Britain there are currently 158 Red Cross trained practitioners operating through 119 hospitals and 23 Red Cross centres. If you are resident outside Britain, it might be worth asking your doctor or local health authority whether any similar services operate in your own locality.

## COSMETIC SURGERY

Cosmetic or 'plastic' surgery first arose as a medical speciality towards the end of the 19th century. Not surprisingly, it was the French (who always seem to lead the way in the development of beauty treatments) who first began to practise – albeit somewhat crudely – many of the initial surgical treatments.

Having read some of the early, and mostly horrific, stories detailing the primitive procedures involved, one cannot help but question the sanity, not to mention the vanity, of any woman who willingly presented her face and body for such torturous treatment. According to one report, the great Victorian beauty, the Duchess of Marlborough, spent almost 20 years of her life having annual injections of paraffin wax in her breasts and nose in order to enlarge the former and refine the latter. Although initially successful, this bizarre form of treatment later proved to be the Duchess's undoing, for not only did the wax eventually cause severe inflammation, but ultimately it also seeped into her lymph glands leading to ulceration. As if that was not bad enough, it was later claimed that when the Duchess sat close to a fire, the bridge of her nose actually slid away. Not surprisingly, this practice soon fell into disuse, but not before this hapless victim of her own vanity was driven insane.

Even members of the British Royal Family have, apparently, not been immune to trying out the odd torturous technique or two in the hope of improving their looks. According to the Russian stage star Vera Lionidovna, Queen Alexandra (wife of Edward VII) allowed a Parisian surgeon to scrape the flesh from her face with a sharp spoon until it was a raw wound. Despite the horrific amount of pain involved, this primitive attempt at dermabrasion was actually said to have resulted in the Princess emerging with such a wonderful new complexion, that many other noble European ladies rushed immediately to Paris in her wake to see what magic could be wrought upon their own faces by this incredible technique.

Mary Pickford, Lady Diana Cooper, Lucille Ball, Carmen Miranda and Tallulah Bankhead were among many who willingly submitted themselves to the surgeon's scalpel when the first clumsy attempts at face-lift surgery became all the rage. Sadly, not all of them were entirely pleased with the results of their surgeon's handiwork.

While we may be tempted to laugh at the lengths to which

some of these early 'guinea pigs' were prepared to go, it is probably true to say that there can be few of us who have not wished, at some point in our lives, to alter our own appearance. Forty or fifty years ago, such a wish would have been destined to remain merely an unfulfilled fantasy for the average person. Apart from the enormous cost involved, the very idea of undergoing surgery in order to improve upon the physical characteristics with which nature had seen fit to endow one would have been regarded as the ultimate in self-indulgence. In those days, vanity was still a dirty word, and even the fortunate and famous few who possessed sufficient money to immunise themselves against the general consensus of opinion were often loathe to acknowledge publicly that they had submitted to the surgeon's scalpel.

Today, both the techniques and the emphasis have changed quite dramatically. Modern society places so much pressure on us all to look as good as we can for as long as we can, that all kinds of people — from politicians, film stars and media celebrities right through to secretaries, housewives, and even students — have happily altered some facet of their physical appearance with cosmetic surgery. And far from being derided for it, society not only applauds such decisions, but actively encourages the rest of us to feel less than satisfied with our own appearance.

With recent advances in technology, it has now become possible to alter virtually any part of your anatomy that you dislike. Heavy ankles and knees can be slimmed down with surgery; fat and flab can be sliced off stomachs, hips, bottoms, or thighs; and breasts can be reduced, resculpted, recontoured, lifted, or enlarged. Chins and noses can be built-up, reshaped or pared down; eyelids can be lifted; bags can be removed; cheekbones can be added to refine the facial features; and thin lips can be plumped up to form what research shows is the sexiest and most alluring of all mouth shapes: a perfect, baby-like pout.

And it is not only women who are taking advantage of the latest range of cosmetic surgery skills. In fact, such are the

wonders that can be created when science, surgery and technology combine, that a whole host of new and innovative
techniques have now been devised to help transform the ordinary, average man into a superman. In addition to enlarging
many a female breast, silicone implants are also now being
employed to provide men with a little bit of extra pecs-appeal;
buttock implants – a hot favourite with gays and transsexuals
– can turn a flat rear end into a tempting pair of nicely rounded
apple dumplings; men who suffer the shame of droopy femi-
nine-like breasts can regain their pride by having fat cells
extracted from their chest; and if they are less than happy with
the girth of their prized appendage, they can kill two birds of
insecurity with one stone by having the fat transferred to where
it will be more appreciated – to pad out the girth of their
penis.

Even more remarkably, men now have the added option of
a super-value three-in-one procedure. In addition to incorporating both above-mentioned techniques, this can also add a
vital extra half to three-quarters of an inch to a man's self-
esteem. According to one American surgeon who offers this
special package deal, an increase in length can be obtained
simply by snipping through a suspensory ligament at the base
of the penis.

Cosmetic surgery has, in fact, become so acceptable,
respectable and widespread that, with a little saving, it is now
within the reach of everyone. Regardless of this, however, one
inescapable fact still remains – altering your appearance with
cosmetic surgery might make you look better on the surface,
but it can never guarantee that any improvement the surgeon
makes will be more than skin deep. For this reason, it is advisable for anyone contemplating such a step to  appraise
*realistically* both what they hope to achieve by altering their
appearance, and also what effect this may or may not have on
their life.

What follows is a list of the latest surgical procedures on
offer, together with a detailed description of what each one
entails. As prices can vary quite considerably between differ-

ent countries, and even between different surgeons and clinics in the same country, individuals considering any of the surgical procedures outlined would be best advised to make their own enquiries and compare the costs offered by a number of *reputable and accredited* surgeons and/or clinics. They should also have satisfactory answers to the following questions before proceeding:

- Is the clinic accredited?
- What are the surgeon's and anaesthetist's qualifications?
- What results can you *realistically* expect?
- Are there any risks involved, and what are they?
- What precisely does the procedure involve? (Remember, you will be committing both your body and a significant sum of money to the enterprise, so you have every right to demand and expect a detailed explanation.)
- For how long will the operation last?
- For how long will you be hospitalised?
- How much pain or discomfort will be involved?
- Will there be any swelling or bruising?
- How long should it take for any scars to heal?
- How long will it be before any stitches are removed?
- How long should it take for you to make a complete recovery?
- What after-care is offered by the surgeon/clinic?
- Are there any special preparations you should make or instructions you should follow prior to the operation?
- What should you do if any complications occur? (And, more to the point, what steps will be taken by the surgeon/clinic in such an instance?)
- What will be the total, overall cost, including the surgeon's and anaesthetist's fees, hospital stay, etc.?
- When is payment expected?
- Can the surgeon put you in touch with any former patients who would be willing to talk to you about their own experience?
- And finally, will there be any cost to you for additional surgery if anything should go wrong?

## Abdominoplasty (Abdominal Skin Tightening)

Not to be confused with an operation to remove fat from the stomach, abdominoplasty can be performed on people of a relatively normal weight whose stomach muscles and abdominal skin have become slackened or overstretched through pregnancy, abdominal surgery, rapid weight loss or previous periods of obesity.

If you are overweight at the time of consultation you will be advised to defer surgery until you have achieved a satisfactory weight loss. If, despite this, a few areas of spot fat still remain, the surgeon may offer to remove this by liposuction when surgery is performed.

Under general anaesthetic, an incision will be made across the lower abdomen, the precise shape of which will be largely determined by such factors as the surgeon's personal preference for surgical technique and the specific nature of the patient's problem. Whichever type of incision is used, the surgeon will take care to conceal the evidence of his or her work within the pubic hair region and the natural body creases formed between the thighs and trunk.

A further incision will be made all around the navel, which will be raised and left attached to its blood supply until the surgeon is ready to slot it into its new position. After separating skin, subcutaneous tissue and spot fat from the underlying musculature, the surgeon will trim any stretched muscle tissue in order to tighten it. The flap of skin will be stretched and pulled down to fit neatly and tautly over the stomach and abdomen, a new site will be excised into which the navel will be slotted and stitched, and the excess skin will be removed prior to suturing the remainder back together again. Suction drains are necessary in order to prevent blood clotting, and the patient is required to remain on her back for the first few days of recovery.

### Hospitalisation Period
Five to seven days.

### Benefits and Claims

A flatter, tighter abdomen and, possibly, the disappearance of any stretch marks or scars that may be apparent in any area from which the excess skin is to be removed.

This procedure is not advisable in the following circumstances:

- Within a year of surgery for gallstones or ulcers.
- If any future pregnancies are intended.
- If you have previously suffered from phlebitis.

### Results

While the results of this operation are usually permanent, there will be a good deal of initial pain and discomfort, especially when walking. Swelling and bruising may last for anything between three and six weeks. Sex is banned for between four and six weeks but, under the circumstances, this would probably be more of a relief than a hardship. The client will have two scars – one in the area of the bikini line; the other around the navel. These may be thin and delicate or thick and lumpy; it all depends upon the type of skin you have, the skill of your surgeon, and whether any complications arise during and/or after surgery. On the whole, however, most people have made a full recovery within six to twelve weeks, at which time you can expect to enjoy all the benefits of having a nice, firm, flat stomach that will look terrific in clothes and, discounting any visible scarring, may even look good out of them as well!

### Potential Complications

As with any form of surgery, there are always risks attached. These could include haemotomas; haemorrhaging; deep-vein thrombosis; infection; a temporary or permanent loss of sensation or numbness in and around the area operated upon if damage is sustained to any of the nerves; and extensive or unsightly scarring.

## Breast Reshaping (Mammoplasty)

As science and society constantly discover new ways to increase and extend the most useful, viable, productive and attractive years of a woman's life, more and more women are turning to surgery in order to either sustain, enhance or improve the statistics that nature and genetics originally endowed them with, and that time, motherhood and gravity are threatening to erode.

Few women are entirely satisfied with the shape, size and overall dimensions of their breasts. The small-breasted usually yearn to be larger; the big-breasted often long to be smaller; while even those whose breasts nestle comfortably in the confines of an average 34 or 36 B-cup will often confess to being dissatisfied with either the volume, the contours, the position or the condition of their breasts.

Breast reshaping can reduce, augment, lift, reshape and realign the breasts. Nipples can be repositioned or corrected if inverted. It is even possible to construct a whole new breast if surgery for cancer results in losing an existing one. Like most forms of surgery, mammoplasty is not entirely without risks, and whilst complaints stemming from breast-reduction or lifting operations are relatively rare, a great deal of controversy still surrounds the use of silicone to enlarge the breasts.

## Breast Augmentation

In theory, breasts can be enlarged to virtually any size, but how far the surgeon is prepared to increase your breast size very much depends on the elasticity of your skin. Unless you have ambitions to look like Brigitte Neilsen, this should not present much of a problem.

Some surgeons like to site the implant just beneath the breast tissue covering the pectoral muscle. Others (and this is more common nowadays) believe it's better to place the prosthesis beneath the pectorals, as this creates a softer and more natural look and feel. The precise location of the incision (and therefore the resulting scar) could be in any one of three places: in the crease beneath the breast; around the areola of the nipple; or under the armpit. As most surgeons have their own preference, this should be discussed in advance.

The operation will take between 1½–2 hours, and small drains will usually be left in place for the following 24 hours to control any bleeding that might occur. Bandages must be worn around the breasts for between five and ten days, and when these are removed, a long-line bra should be worn night and day for at least three weeks to provide support.

Your breasts will obviously be very painful for the first few days, but this usually starts to diminish from around the third day. Lifting, stretching and other extended arm movements are banned for the first week or so, and you will be advised not to drive, as friction from the seat belts could make your breasts sore. Any swelling caused by the surgery (though not that caused by the implant!) should subside within three to six weeks, after which time you can resume your normal lifestyle. Some surgeons recommend massaging the breasts for at least five minutes, three or four times daily, in order to help prevent any hardening of surrounding breast tissue.

### Hospitalisation Period
One to two nights.

### Benefits and Claims
All the obvious ones.

### Results
There will be a scar which, depending on its location, may or may not be visible; the least noticeable are those resulting from incisions made around the nipple. As only around six per cent of women opt to have their implants removed, we must suppose that even those who do experience some problems with contracture (hardening, when fibrous scars form in the surrounding breast tissue) would rather stick with their implants than live with smaller breasts.

## Potential Complications

Around one in three breast enlargement operations usually result in some degree of contracture. The risk of post-operative infection is low (about one per cent), but if this does occur, then the implants should be removed, and not replaced until antibiotics have completely cured the problem.

Rumours of implants exploding aboard aeroplanes are without foundation, but implants filled with saline (rather than gel) have been known to rupture suddenly, which can be an embarrassing, and rather deflating, experience, and all types of implants currently in use are vulnerable to leakage.

Finally, while some specialists deny that the risk of developing cancer is any greater in women with breast implants, there is some evidence to suggest that implants might make it more difficult to detect its existence.

## Breast-lifting

Age, gravity, breastfeeding and a significant reduction in weight can all cause loss of elasticity and subsequent drooping of the breasts. While sagging, droopy breasts can be corrected surgically, any uplifting effect is not a permanent cure for the 'landslide effect' of age. When this is considered together with the fact that any form of surgical incursion into the body inevitably results in scars, this type of corrective surgery seems less advisable and far less attractive to the consumer.

As most breast-lifting operations only involve removing a section of stretched, excess skin in order to raise the position of the breasts, the procedure itself is fairly simple. (If the breasts are very small to begin with, it is possible for an implant to be inserted at the same time to augment their size.) The technique is similar to that described for breast-reduction with the nipple and areola being repositioned, but as no living tissue is excised, the duration of the operation is shorter. While the recovery period is similar to that outlined for the breast-reduction procedure, patients usually experience far less post-operative swelling, discomfort and pain.

### Benefits and Claims

The operation is supposed to raise the position of the breasts so that they sit higher on the chest. This sometimes results in a recontouring of the overall shape. Any stretch marks apparent in the excised skin will be removed, but not those that exist elsewhere on the breast.

### Hospitalisation Period

Two days.

### Results

Although this type of surgery can undoubtedly make the breasts look more youthful and shapely, the result will only be a temporary one as time and gravity will still continue to exert their effects. How long the effects of this operation last depends on a number of factors, including the elasticity of your skin; how much weight you gain or lose in the intervening period; and whether any future pregnancies (and breast-feeding) occur.

### Potential Complications

These are similar to those that can arise following breast-reduction. As the nipple is rarely detached before being resited, however, there are fewer problems and risks attached to lifting the breasts than reducing their overall size.

## Breast Reconstruction

The question of whether or not to include breast reconstruction in a book of beauty treatments was a difficult one to resolve. Strictly speaking, this particular procedure is not one that is ever likely to be considered by, or offered to, any woman who is merely dissatisfied with the size or shape of her existing breasts.

On reflection, however, I felt it was worth including, if only for the fact that it may provide some useful information for any woman who has been unfortunate enough to lose a breast due to cancer. For putting aside the vanity factor and the question of individual preferences for body size and shape, there cannot be anything more devastating to a woman's psychological well-being than to face life – even a life that is all the more precious for having beaten cancer – without a breast.

Out of all the possible surgical techniques that are available to augment the female breast, reconstructing a breast that has become damaged by, or lost completely to, cancer must be the most skilful, satisfying and rewarding of all cosmetic operations a surgeon could be asked to perform, while the benefits to the patient must be inestimable.

There are a variety of methods for reconstructing a breast. One traditional technique involves removing and transferring skin and tissue from another area of the body, such as the back or the abdomen, and, if necessary, supplementing this with a synthetic prosthesis. More recently, however, a new technique has been devised utilising the skin's natural ability to stretch. This involves inserting a temporary implant beneath the skin at the site of the new breast. A connecting tube is attached to the implant and left in place for a period of time during which a saline solution is repeatedly inserted. This acts to pump up the breast thereby causing the skin surrounding the inflatable sac to stretch gradually until it attains the appropriate size. The sac and feeder tube are then removed and the new breast is ready for the implantation of a silicone gel prosthesis or body fat and tissue.

Although it is feasible that a new breast could be reconstructed during a mastectomy operation, or soon afterwards, many surgeons prefer to wait for at least six months in order to ensure there is no recurrence of the cancer. In cases where radiotherapy or chemotherapy treatment follows mastectomy, reconstruction of the breast is not advisable until at least 12 months have passed. As statistics show that four out of every five cases of recurrence are likely to show up within the first year, this can be a wise precaution.

As with other breast operations, there will be considerable swelling, bruising and soreness for several weeks. Arm movements will be painful and restricted, but this will gradually diminish as recovery takes place. Other details of post-operative pain, care and recovery will be similar to those outlined in the section on breast augmentation.

### Benefits and Claims

The emotional and psychological benefits of breast-reconstruction surgery can be so great they are virtually impossible to quantify. The fact that this type of surgery affords the only means for many female cancer victims to resume anything approaching a near-normal life makes it well worth considering, as the end result could far outweigh any of the potential risks involved.

### Hospitalisation Period

Ten to twelve days.

### Results

Some women who have this operation are adamant about recreating as realistic a breast as possible, while others just want a reasonable facsimile that will pass unnoticed in swimsuits and clothes. If you belong to the former group, then you will obviously need to have further surgery to reconstruct a nipple and areola. These can be made by taking a skin graft from the remaining nipple, the genitals, the ear lobe, or the inside of the upper thigh, but you will have to wait for around three months so that the surgeon can be sure that the new breast is healing well, and that there are unlikely to be any problems with poor blood supply to the new nipple and areola. As the actual grafting can be completed within an hour, and can be carried out under a local anaesthetic, an overnight stay will not be necessary.

Although scarring can be extensive, both around the breast and in the area from which fat and tissue has been transferred, many women are so delighted with their new breast(s) that they are only too happy to disregard these.

## Potential Complications

Muscle and tissue can atrophy and die if damaged is sustained to the blood supply. The risk of tissue dying has been estimated at around three per cent in cases where muscle is moved from the back to the chest, and anything up to 30 per cent when it is moved from the abdomen. Further complications can arise when liquefied fat taken from the abdomen oozes out of the breast. Apart from being uncomfortable and unpleasant, this can also result in a subsequent loss of volume and consequently the overall size of the new breast.

The formation of blood clots at the site where fat and muscle have been removed from the back are fairly common, although the risk of this occurring can be minimised or prevented by leaving the drainage tubes in place for a longer period. Other risks include infection, loss of sensation and lack of symmetry between the old and new breast.

## Breast Reduction

For every small-breasted woman who hankers after larger breasts, there is likely to be a large-breasted woman who would give anything to swap places with her. Despite the admiring glances they often elicit, large breasts can be an acutely embarrassing nuisance. Apart from the fact that many people insist on adhering unkindly to the notion that the size of a woman's brain is in inverse proportion to the size of her breasts, they can also place severe restrictions on a woman's activities. Moreover, breasts that are seriously over-large can cause so much physical discomfort and strain, that the idea of having them reduced is perceived as being more of a blessed relief than a stressful surgical ordeal.

As reducing the size of the breasts involves removing a quantity of breast tissue and repositioning the nipples, the operation itself can be quite involved, often taking up to three hours. Depending on the size of the existing breast and how much tissue is to be removed, the nipple will either be removed completely and then regrafted on to the breast; or, as in the breast-enlargement operation, it may be left attached to the stalk containing its blood supply and nerve endings and simply slotted into its new site once the excess tissue has been removed.

Post-operative pain and swelling can be quite considerable for the first 48 hours or so. Once the drainage tubes have been removed and you are allowed to return home, however, any discomfort should gradually diminish, but it may take a few weeks for swelling to subside and for the final new size of the breasts to be apparent. All other aspects of post-operative care and recovery are the same as those outlined in the breast-enlargement section.

### Benefits and Claims
The operation leads to smaller breasts and, in some cases, a slight improvement in their shape. Further benefits include less restriction, fewer backaches and greater freedom of movement.

### Hospitalisation Period
Two to three days.

### Results
This operation has a high satisfaction rating – one of the highest, in fact, of all breast surgery. The majority of women who opt for breast reduction are only too happy to swap their heavy, pendulous breasts for a smaller, lighter bosom, considering any scars they sustain in the process – and these can be quite extensive – well worth it.

### Potential Complications
There is a one-in-ten chance of developing hard, tender lumps and bumps which are often mistaken for cancer. Whilst these can cause some alarm and distress, they are in fact nothing more serious than lumps of fat which have become hardened due to inefficient blood circulation immediately following surgery. Although they will disappear, this could take anything

up to six months, and sometimes even longer. Other complications include a loss of sensation in one or both nipples and, in very rare cases, loss of the nipple itself, should severe post-operative restriction in the blood supply fail to right itself.

## Cheek Implantation

Many people are envious of those with well-defined, highly placed cheekbones. Apart from giving interest and definition to the shape of the face, high cheekbones can help provide additional support to ageing, droopy facial skin. On the whole, however, relatively few people dislike their own features so much that they are prepared to change the entire shape and look of their face by having their cheeks surgically augmented.

The people most likely to be attracted to this form of cosmetic surgery are those whose looks are important to their career, such as actors, actresses, models and singers. Members of certain ethnic groups, such as the Chinese, sometimes wish to adopt a more 'Westernised' appearance.

As cheek implantation is a relatively simple procedure that rarely takes more than an hour, surgery can be performed under local anaesthetic on an out-patient basis. An incision will be made from inside the mouth high up in the area covering the underlying structure of the cheekbone. The outer layers of skin and muscle will be separated from the underlying layers to form a pocket into which the silicone gel implant will be placed. Once everything has been sutured back into place, strips of bandage will be taped across the cheeks to help keep swelling to a minimum, and to hold the implant firmly in position while the healing process takes place.

Although this is not regarded as a particularly painful procedure, there will be some stiffness, numbness and bruising of the mouth and cheeks for a while. This will make normal activities such as laughing, eating and talking uncomfortable and difficult for a period, but this should gradually diminish after a week or so. It will, however, mean that you will not be allowed to chew any solid food or clean your teeth until the wound inside the mouth has begun to heal. Regular mouth rinses of salt water will help speed up healing as well as minimise any risk of infection.

Although you should be able to return to work after about a week, all forms of vigorous sport, or exercise involving facial muscles (such as singing and playing a musical instrument with your mouth) will be vetoed until the cheeks have healed. Unfortunately, sex and kissing will also be banned for at least two weeks.

### Benefits and Claims

The flatter your natural face and cheekbones, the more pronounced any visual difference will be after implants have been inserted.

### Results

Providing there are no complications, the results are usually permanent, and as the scars will be on the inside of the cheek, evidence of the operation will not be visible.

### Potential Complications

The risk of infection is low, though this is greater for smokers than non-smokers. If you are unfortunate enough to contract an infection, the implant will need to be removed for the duration of treatment and then reinserted. Numbness of the cheeks and upper lip can occur, but this usually disappears within a few weeks or months.

Other, less common, problems include one of the implants slipping out of place, or leakage and deflation caused by injury or a hard knock to the cheek or face.

## Chin Correction (Mentoplasty)

Reducing an over-large chin that juts out, or building up one that recedes are considered to be relatively easy, safe and trouble-free procedures. It is only when realignment of the jaw and teeth are involved that it becomes much more time-consuming, complex and intricate, and is classed as a major operation.

There are two main techniques for correcting a receding chinline. One involves a silicone implant; the other involves realigning the bones and then wiring them into their new position. As both techniques can be carried out via an incision made inside the mouth, any scarring will be invisible. With chin-reduction procedures, surgery is also usually carried out through the mouth, with the excess bone being chiselled or planed away and the chin remodelled into a more refined, less prominent shape.

Swelling and bruising of the lower half of the face is inevitable. In some cases this may also extend to the lips. Any pain and discomfort will be minimised by keeping still and avoiding facial movements. Post-operative care and recovery details are the same as for cheek augmentation.

## Benefits and Claims
Chin correction improves the shape and definition of the chin and jawline, and rebalances the overall features to give a more 'normal', refined effect.

## Hospitalisation Period
One to two days.

## Results
Usually very good and, barring any complications, the results will be permanent.

## Potential Complications
The risks associated with chin augmentation are fairly low. As with any operation, infection can occur; if it does, the implant will have to be removed and reinserted when the infection has been cured. Blows to the chin can cause implants to leak or slip out of place, either of which is likely to result in further surgery to correct the problem.

With chin-reduction procedures there is some risk to the

nerves which may sustain damage during surgery. This can result in a degree of numbness and loss of sensation for a period of weeks, months and even up to a year. Swelling, which may not be immediately apparent to others, can last for several months. As might be expected, the risk of developing infection is higher for smokers than non-smokers.

## Collagen Injections

Within the dermis, which is found beneath the outer layers of the skin, lies a network of interwoven fibres. These are made up of a protein substance called collagen which acts as a foundation to support the entire structure of the skin. It is collagen's ability to retain water that gives the skin its smooth, plump contours and supple elasticity. With age and time, however, this network of collagen fibres gradually weakens. As the fibres lose their ability to hold water, they begin to harden and shift position. This degeneration of supportive tissue – which is hastened by such factors as over-exposure to natural and artificial sunlight, smoking, poor diet, inadequate exercise and airborne pollution – causes areas of depression to form which then show up on the skin's surface as wrinkles, furrows, lines and crow's feet.

Collagen injections could be described as a form of under-pinning for the face in so far as they act like a temporary support for a weakened structure. A highly purified form of bovine collagen is injected into areas that are beginning to show signs of collapse, such as facial grooves, lines and wrinkles. These areas can, in a manner of speaking, be propped up and filled out to give an appearance of plumper, smoother and younger-looking, relatively wrinkle-free skin.

As this treatment must be avoided if you suffer from certain medical conditions, such as rheumatoid arthritis, it is important to advise your practitioner of your medical history at the time of consultation. A sensitivity test should also be taken before undergoing collagen injections. This involves injecting a minute quantity of collagen into the forearm at least 28 days before treatment and then monitoring the area to see if any adverse reaction is experienced.

The actual procedure, which is claimed to be relatively painless, takes around an hour. After applying an anaesthetic cream to the relevant area, the surgeon injects collagen (mixed with a local anaesthetic) just beneath the skin into the fold of the line or wrinkle. Despite claims to the contrary, however, injections in or near sensitive areas like the mouth and nostrils may often cause a sharp, stinging sensation – so do be prepared to experience some degree of discomfort (precisely how much will depend upon your pain threshold).

The skin around the area injected will swell up, and may redden or bruise slightly, but this should subside within 48 hours. However, as several sessions are usually recommended to achieve the best results, it is best to prepare yourself for an uncomfortable few weeks.

## Benefits and Claims

Collagen treatments produce smoother, plumper-looking facial skin, and a temporary 'lifting' of expression lines, furrows, wrinkles, crow's feet and small lines that radiate from the upper lip. Injections may also help 'fill in' small scars resulting from acne and chickenpox, but are not suitable for the deeper 'pitted' type of acne scar depression. Thin lips can be enlarged with collagen injections, and this is popular with models and actresses seeking the bee-stung-lip look.

## Results

Although collagen injections can be extremely effective at eradicating deep lines and furrows, they are not a permanent panacea because the collagen eventually gets absorbed by the body. Effects rarely last beyond two years and, on some skins, as little as six months depending on how well your skin reacts. Moreover, as many people have proved to be allergic to the substance, they are not suitable for everyone. When used in conjunction with a face lift, however, they can provide the extra finishing touch to any areas where the surgery has been not quite so effective.

Collagen injections are considerably cheaper than surgery, but the price could still knock a hefty hole in the average woman's pocket. Given the transitory nature of its effects, it is worth weighing up very carefully *all* the pros and cons before going ahead.

## Cosmetic Face Peeling

Whilst this is classified as a *non-surgical* procedure, it is still necessary for patients to be sedated for an hour or so while the special skin-peeling solution is applied to their face. Once this has been accomplished, the face will be kept covered with bandages for 48 hours. When the surgical tape is removed, it takes with it the old crepy layers of epidermal skin. A special surgical powder is then applied to help dry and protect the new skin. Over the next five days, the patient is encouraged to take plenty of facial showers in order to help remove the dried powder.

### Hospitalisation Period
Seven days.

### Benefits and Claims
The aim of face-peeling is to renew the supportive structure of the skin and reduce age lines and wrinkles. As this is recommended for those with mature skin, many surgeons will not accept patients below the age of 40. However, it is said to be suitable also for faces that have been left with severe skin scarring from acne, but only after all outbreaks have ceased.

The chemical solution penetrates the outer layers of the skin (the epidermis) into the dermal layer where it acts to rearrange the collagen and elastic fibres and give the skin a more youthful tightness, elasticity and support. The peeling solution is also said to have a secondary effect in that it removes the top layers of the epidermis, thereby encouraging the skin cells to produce new baby-soft skin.

What actually happens, in effect, is that the chemical solution destroys the outer layer of the skin by a process that amounts literally to burning. As happens with any form of burn, the skin will then peel off to expose the underlying tissue, thereby forcing the growth of new skin. Not surprisingly, therefore, this procedure could involve some considerable discomfort and pain, and will undoubtedly have a pretty frightening effect on your appearance during the early stages of recovery. As the healing process takes place, the skin will itch badly, but it is very important not to scratch it as this could damage the tender new skin that will be forming.

## Results

Initially the skin will take on a rosy pink or perhaps even a scarlet hue, rather as if it has been over-exposed to the sun. This could last for anything between six to twelve weeks, during which time great care should be taken to keep it clean and well moisturised. It is also important to avoid exposing your face to the elements, as this could result in blotchiness and uneven pigmentation. For the first few weeks, your skin may also appear rather grainy in texture, but this should return to normal after about four weeks or so.

Whilst this is a painful and very inconvenient facial rejuvenation process, there is no doubt that chemical peeling can remove many (but not necessarily all) of the surface lines and wrinkles that contribute to an ageing appearance. Results with acne sufferers have shown a noticeable reduction in acne-scar tissue, and smoother, softer skin texture. Patients are advised not to wear any make up for at least two weeks, and then only non-allergenic brands.

## Potential Complications

As a general rule, chemical peeling works best on paler skins. Olive complexions have a tendency towards blotchiness and irregular pigmentation following chemical peeling, while it is not recommended at all for black and oriental skins. If you are unsure how your skin might react, ask for a patch test to be done and then monitor the result for at least four weeks before making your decision.

Complications can include prolonged redness, increased sensitivity to the sun, a permanent change in pigmentation and the formation of small, raised scars.

## Ear Correction (Otoplasty)

Abnormally prominent ears (sometimes unkindly referred to as 'bat ears') can be the cause of much misery and distress to their owners. The ears are usually fully grown by the age of six, so any deformity of size will be evident in childhood. As children of this age are not noted for their tact and subtlety, young sufferers can have a wretchedly unhappy time. Once they reach adolescence, they usually seek surgery of their own accord.

Quite often, otoplasty can be very successful in both correcting the angle at which the ears protrude from the skull and also at reducing the apparent size of the ear. In most cases, the apparent deformity is caused by an oversized conchal bowl (the large central depression within the ear) and a small or poorly defined ear fold, which is the part that looks rather like a shell.

Surgery usually takes between one and two hours for each ear. It can be performed under local or general anaesthetic (with very young children a general anaesthetic is advisable in order to prevent them becoming distressed or wriggling around). An incision is made in the crease behind the ear and the skin is separated from the cartilage. The surgeon then trims down the cartilage and any excess tissue and, if necessary, the remaining cartilage is re–sculpted or modified to give a more shell-like appearance around the inner ear. The size of the conchal bowl is then reduced and the ears are 'pinned back' by being stitched very carefully in position so that they lay more flatly against the side of the head. When operating on the second ear, special care is taken to ensure that both ears are closely matched in size and position.

Patients are usually allowed home the same day. The ears are protected with heavy padding which is secured by bandages wrapped around the head. These should remain in place for between five and seven days, but some form of head-covering will have to be worn at night for the first few weeks in order to prevent the ears being crushed or folded whilst sleeping.

There will be considerable swelling and discomfort, and some short-term pain but, barring any problems, this should subside significantly after a few days. Children are able to return to school, and adults to work, after seven days, but swimming should be avoided for the first week or two, and any other form of exercise that may result in injury to the ears should be avoided for a further two months. The ears will probably be fairly numb for some time and could remain sensitive to extremes of heat and cold for anything up to a year.

## Results

Although the scars will be fairly long (between two and three inches), they are concealed within the crease behind the ear so there should be no problem with visibility. Providing there are no post-operative complications, the results, which in most cases are highly satisfactory, will be permanent.

## Potential Complications

Although this operation carries a low risk of infection, this will be enhanced if the ear has sustained any injuries prior to surgical correction. If an infection should occur, it is vital to seek medical attention immediately. If left untreated, infections can result in permanent damage to the cartilage or some deformity in appearance. A course of antibiotics should be prescribed without delay if you experience any of the following: severe, continuous pain for more than 48 hours; bleeding; or any significant increase (rather than a decrease) in reddening or swelling of the ear within the first few days following surgery.

There is some risk of swelling due to the formation of blood clots, but these can be easily treated by draining off any excess blood that collects beneath the surface of the ear. Sores can develop within the bowl or shell-like area of the ear, but as these are often caused by the pressure of dressings, leaving the ears uncovered should result in a quick cure. Some movement can occur in the positioning of one or both ears due to failure of the stitches to hold the ears firmly in place.

## Eyelid and Eye Bag Correction (Blepharoplasty)

Especially popular with middle-aged men, blepharoplasty is probably one of the simplest and most frequently performed cosmetic operations. Although some people find 'heavy-lidded' eyes (à la Robert Mitchum and Marlene Deitrich) exceedingly sensual and attractive, many people who develop droopy eyelids and sagging bags in middle–age often regard their presence as unattractive and uncomfortable reminders of their rapidly advancing years.

A person's lids will occasionally droop so badly over the eyes that his or her vision becomes partly obscured. Regardless of whether the cause is genetic, or the result of a problem with the thyroid gland, the only solution in such cases is to have the eyelids corrected surgically before the muscles become so over-stretched that an operation to support the eyelids becomes too complicated to perform.

Before pursuing blepharoplasty it is important to note the following:

1) As puffiness and swelling around the eyes is symptomatic in some illnesses, do have a thorough check-up with your doctor first.
2) Blepharoplasty will not cure excessively dark circles beneath the eyes.
3) It is not recommended for those who suffer with 'dry-eye' syndrome.

Surgery to correct the upper eyelids can be performed under a general or local anaesthetic. It is a simpler procedure than lower-eyelid surgery, and it rarely takes more than an hour to complete. The incision is made either in the arc formed by the natural crease of the upper eyelid, or close to the eyelash line. Having peeled back the outer layer of skin, the surgeon will then remove any excess skin, tissue and underlying fat before suturing the remaining skin back into position.

Surgery to remove under-eye bags is a little more complex, and therefore requires more care and greater technical skill. As it is difficult to judge precisely how much skin should be trimmed, some surgeons prefer to use a local anaesthetic so that the patient can remain awake with their eyes open through-out the operation. Alternatively, if you find this too distressing to contemplate, the surgeon will carry out the operation under general anaesthetic using an assistant to hold your eyes open. The actual procedure is the same as that outlined for upper-eyelid surgery, except that in this instance the incision will be made close to the eyelash line on the lower lid.

Neither procedure requires an overnight stay in hospital. The dressings are fairly minimal – just enough to cover and protect the stitches. Your eyelids will feel sore and ache imme-diately afterwards, and there will be some degree of swelling or redness and bruising for the first week, and perhaps longer if the skin on your eyelids is particularly delicate or sensitive. Applying cold packs to the eyes will help reduce any swelling and bruising.

As swelling of the eyelids can cause interference with tear drainage, any overnight stickiness and crusting needs to be thor-oughly cleansed away on rising. This can be accomplished with the aid of moistened cotton buds. As the healing process takes place, this problem should gradually diminish and disappear altogether after the first week. Sunglasses are recommended to protect the eyes as they will remain sensitive to the sun, strong artificial light, smoke, dust and airborne pollution for anything up to a month. Contact-lens wearers will have to make do with spectacles for the first fortnight, and eye make-up should be avoided for at least the first seven days.

Normal social activities can be resumed after a week. As

extra care must be taken in any situation involving physical contact, sex is best avoided for at least another week, and any form of competitive sport will be banned for several weeks more.

## Results
Scarring should be minimal, and mostly concealed within the upper and lower creases of the eyelids. The overall effect, which can last for up to 10 years, will be of a dramatic revitalisation of the face without it being apparent that you have had surgery. The eyes will look younger, less tired and far more lively and alert.

## Potential Complications
As skin in this area usually heals very well, the risks and complications are relatively few. Those that do occur are more likely with under-eye surgery, where the greatest risk is of the surgeon removing too much skin resulting in a wide-eyed staring look, or 'pop-eyes'. Sometimes, this problem will correct itself as the skin and muscle gradually stretch to become more supple and elastic. In severe cases, however, skin grafting may be the only cure.

Other potential problems include a lack of symmetry between the eyes; the removal of too much fat, which can result in a sunken-eyed look; a slight impairment to vision; and, in extremely rare cases, blindness.

## Dermabrasion

As with cosmetic peeling, dermabrasion aims to improve the appearance of the skin by surgically removing the top layer in the hope that the underlying layers will heal and grow through more smoothly. The only difference is that where cosmetic peeling relies on a chemical substance to gradually 'burn' or lift off the upper layers of skin over a period of days, dermabrasion achieves this instantly with the aid of a power-operated device to which a wire brush or stone abrader is attached. If

you have ever watched someone sanding down brick or paint-
work you will have a fairly good idea of how this seemingly
gruesome technique works, and why most surgeons prefer to
do it under general anaesthetic.

If a large area of the face is to be abraded, it is usual for
the surgeon to do a patch test at the first session, then wait
for a few months to see how well the skin responds and to
assess whether there is likely to be any significant alteration
in pigmentation. If the results are good, dermabrasion of the
area to be treated will take place, after which a final 'improving' session will follow six or twelve months later.

Each session should last around an hour, and as there can
be extensive bleeding, both during and after the operation,
antibiotic ointments and medicated bandages will be applied
to the areas treated. Although this procedure is not especially
painful, it does often result in a considerable amount of
swelling. Apart from the obvious discomfort this can cause, it
will make talking, eating and drinking difficult for the first
few days.

Some surgeons like to remove the bandages themselves a
day or two after the operation; others prefer to leave them in
place for around five days, after which they will either simply
fall away, or become so loose that you can easily peel them
off yourself. However, if the bandaging has not come loose
by the beginning of the second week, medical assistance should
be sought.

You can expect to be off work, and out of the public eye,
for at least 10 days, as it will probably take at least that long
for your face to lose its resemblance to something out of a
horror movie and start returning to normal. Once you have
passed this milestone, your initial reaction to your reflection
will probably be one of delight. Do bear in mind, however,
that the swelling (which often persists for anything up to a
month) could be adding an illusory smoothness that may diminish somewhat once your skin has eventually settled down. The
skin will also remain sensitive, tender and slightly rosy in
colour for six to twelve months, so do avoid the sun as much

as possible, and whenever you can you should wear sunblock and a hat to shield your skin from the sun's damaging rays.

### Results
Although it is not quite as effective as cosmetic peeling at smoothing out wrinkles, dermabrasion often yields better results in treating the deeper pits and depressions that can result from acne flare-ups and chickenpox. It can also improve the appearance of some scars resulting from earlier facial cuts and accidents, or previous surgery. However, neither dermabrasion nor cosmetic peeling are particularly effective at removing the very deep type of scars that are commonly known as 'ice-pick' scars.

### Potential Complications
Although true infection is rare with this type of procedure, the skin may often appear as if it has become infected. Other risks include permanent alteration in the pigment of some areas of the skin, and the formation of small, white spots (which can be treated if they do not disappear on their own). Some people have shown a tendency to develop small, raised scars, but as this is often revealed by the initial patch test it can be fairly safely assumed that your surgeon would not have advised completing the procedure if your own risk factor had been high.

## Face-lift (Rhytidectomy)

Time and gravity take their toll on everyone's appearance. For reasons of heredity, some people may fare better than others by retaining a younger-looking appearance for longer, but sooner or later, a gradual diminution in muscle tone and loss of skin elasticity is bound to affect us all.

Just like a candle that is beginning to melt, once the underlying network of supportive tissue beneath the skin begins to weaken, the flesh covering our bone structure will become increasingly loose and flaccid. By the time we reach our mid-

40s or 50s, many of us will certainly ponder, if not seriously consider, the possibilities and advantages of a face-lift.

A surgical face-lift can be likened to tailoring an over-large garment to fit your body in so far as it involves the surgical removal of excess baggy, facial skin. Unlike the face-lifts of yesteryear, however, which involved smoothing out and stretching the skin across the features and then snipping away the excess, today's advanced techniques pay as much attention to what lies beneath the skin (i.e. muscle, tissue and fat distribution) as they do to its surface. This results in an overall rejuvenation of all the facial features that is far more effective and also far more natural in appearance.

In a full face-lift, the surgeon will correct the forehead and eye area, as well as tighten up any loose folds of skin around the cheeks, jowls, jaw and neck areas. In a half face-lift only the top or bottom half of the face will be attended to. Depending on its complexity, the actual procedure will take between one and two hours.

A face-lift involves an incision being made in the scalp. This will run down in front of the ear, curve round and beneath the lobe and then upward to finish a little way back behind the ear where it will be hidden by the hair. If the forehead is to be included, another incision will be made running from the top of the ear, across the top of the skull to the other ear. This also will be positioned far enough back on the scalp to be undetectable, unless the patient has a problem with receding hair.

Underlying muscle tissue is tightened and trimmed; any excess fat is removed or redistributed; and the skin is smoothed, stretched, trimmed and resewn. The drainage tubes that will have been inserted and the bandaging will remain in place for around 48 hours. Providing there are no complications, the patient will be allowed to return home to convalesce once the bandages and drainage tube have been removed.

Although the stitches will be removed some time between seven and ten days following the operation, it can take anything from two to four weeks for the post-operative swelling and bruising to subside to the point where you feel comfortable in public. It will take at least six months for your muscles to regain their flexibility and your face to settle into its new contours.

### Hospitalisation Period
Two days.

### Benefits and Claims
A surgical face-lift will not stop the hands of time, but it can serve as a delaying mechanism by rewinding them backwards by five or ten years, and sometimes even more. While it is very effective for sagging skin and jowling, and may also smooth out and soften the appearance of deep furrows, it will not erase lines and wrinkles. To remove these, cosmetic peeling would be required or, if your skin is younger, collagen implantation might be a better course.

### Results
Apart from a more youthful physical appearance, there is also a psychological benefit in terms of increased confidence and self-esteem which, in turn, can enhance the effects of the operation. Depending on the quality and texture of your skin, and how well you look after your 'new' face, results can last for five to ten years.

### Potential Complications
Permanent damage or disfigurement is rare nowadays, especially at the hands of a skilled surgeon. As with any form of surgery, however, there are risks. Two of the most common problems are slow or inefficient healing of scar tissue, and haematomas, which occur when blood vessels leak to form clots beneath the skin. In the case of the latter, immediate treatment should be sought as small haematomas can cause the formation of surface lumps which, if not attended to, can take months to disappear, whilst large ones will need to be drained.

Other, and thankfully less common, complications can

include skin sloughing along the scar; sensory nerve damage leading to numbness and loss of sensation; and temporary numbness or paralysis if one of the motor nerves should become damaged during the operation.

## Fat-transferral

Redistributing a person's body fat from one area which has an excess, to other areas that could do with a little more, is fast becoming one of the most popular cosmetic-surgery techniques. Born out of liposuction, fat-transferral sounds like it was invented in response to every woman's – and also many men's – dream of improving their body shape. In many respects it certainly appears – theoretically, at least – to be a logical solution; apart from solving any difficulties inherent in introducing foreign tissue or substances into the body, it also neatly solves the problem of what to do with the fat once it has been removed.

Like most aesthetic techniques, however, fat-transferral is not entirely without its disadvantages. It is not recommended for breast enlargements, which may disappoint many women who have been frightened off by all the recent scare stories about silicone implants. The main reason for this is that fat cells which have been transferred may present signs of calcification – the formation of little lumps that can confuse mammography scans and cause unnecessary alarm.

Under local anaesthetic the surgeon will make a small incision in a fold of skin at the site from where the fat is to be removed. A special enzyme will then be introduced into the area in order to liquefy the fat, and a cannula coupled to a high vacuum chamber – a device somewhat akin to a vacuum cleaner with a long, thin syringe attached – will be inserted to aspirate (suck out) the liquefied fat. The fat is then washed carefully with a saline solution two or three times under sterile conditions in order to filter it, before it is reintroduced into another area.

Fat-transferral is a useful alternative in cases where patients have a proven sensitivity to collagen injections. It can be used to eliminate deeply etched lines between the eyebrows, nose-to-mouth depression lines, scars, crow's feet, sunken cheeks and hollows in the contours of the face. It can also be used to help provide a rounder, perkier look to flat bottoms.

In the United States, fat-transferral is fast emerging as one of the most popular and frequently requested operations to reverse the signs of ageing. This is largely because it is the first method to be discovered that can successfully tackle all the tell-tale areas that have traditionally given away a person's true age. By combining a face lift with fat transferral to plump up the backs of bony, veined hands, fill out sunken cheeks and redefine the contours of the backs of legs when muscle wastage has left them looking scrawny, even octogenarians are discovering that it is now possible to preserve an illusion of greater youth and extend their visual 'shelf life' way beyond all previous expectations.

Depending on the areas to be treated, the procedure takes approximately one-and-a-half hours. As this is performed under a local anaesthetic, an overnight stay is not normally required. Post-operative pain and discomfort should be minimal. Pressure bandages will be applied to the areas treated to keep the 'new' fat in place. If a large area, such as the bottom, has been resculpted or had fat injected to smooth out any dimpling caused by cellulite, a corset-like garment will have to be worn for several days. If the cheeks have been recontoured with fat cells taken from other areas, special facial splints may have to be worn for the first two or three days. Any bruising and swelling should subside within two weeks. A second appointment is usually required after three months to inspect the area and, if necessary, 'top up' the previous treatment with additional fat cells.

### Results

As this technique involves using very fine syringes, no visible scarring should result. As some of the fat is absorbed very quickly, however, the surgeon has to compensate for this by overcorrecting by as much as 50 per cent the area to be augmented with fat cells. This could result in an initially satis-factory appearance that gradually becomes less pleasing as more cells become reabsorbed into the body. Some experts say that anything up to 84 per cent of the fact could be reabsorbed within three years, but that the remaining percentage will survive indefinitely. Others claim that the long-term results are excellent.

### Potential Complications

Injecting too much new fat too close to the skin's surface can result in uneven puckering. If too much fat becomes reab-sorbed in a small area, such as the cheeks, this can cause the formation of uneven 'hill and valley' areas. Infections are rare. Depending on the amount and rate of reabsorption, this proce-dure might need to be repeated every three years in order to build up to the effect you ultimately want.

## Laser Treatment

As our knowledge of the laser beam, and the uses to which it can safely be put increases, laser technology is proving to be a worthy and successful alternative to the scalpel in the treat-ment of a variety of skin-related disorders. Age spots, moles, birthmarks, tattoos and areas of uneven skin pigmentation have all responded well to treatment with specially designed lasers. Research is currently being undertaken to develop its use as a suitable alternative to dermabrasion and chemical peels in cases where the subject may be especially prone to scarring and uneven pigmentation.

In London, treatment with a special pigment lesion laser has been carried out successfully at the Wellington Hospital's Plastic and Reconstructive Surgery Unit. Specifically designed to destroy areas of abnormal superficial skin pigmentation with minimal scarring, the pigment lesion laser uses a wavelength of light that has been carefully selected to maximise absorp-tion by the melanosomes (pigmented structures) whilst minimising the effects on the normal cells and blood vessels surrounding them.

The laser light is delivered in short pulses that treat an area of skin approximately 5 mm in radius. As the laser light is geared to penetrate to only a short depth, this form of treatment is suitable only for superficially pigmented lesions. The best results so far have been obtained in treating freckles, flat pigmented moles, and *café au lait* patches on the skin. As laser treatment generally involves little pain, and only a minimum of discomfort (the sensation is similar to that experienced when an elastic band is pinged against the skin) anaesthetic is rarely required.

Before undergoing laser treatment, patients are advised to avoid exposing to the sun any areas of skin that are to be treated. If the patient has a suntan, treatment will be delayed until it has faded. The use of aspirin prior to treatment should also be avoided, as this can increase the likelihood of local bruising afterwards. However, if aspirin is regularly prescribed to help thin the blood, or the patient is receiving other anti-coagulant therapy or drugs, laser treatment is not advisable.

Following treatment, the areas affected will initially form white patches. In some cases, these may crust over; in many others, they may heal without forming any scabs. Minor crusts or scabs can be treated topically with a mild antiseptic or antibiotic cream. There may be some localised redness and bruising, but this is usually transient with any discolourations fading between seven and fourteen days. Vigorous rubbing or towelling should be avoided after bathing or showering, and shaving is best not attempted until any inflammation has fully settled down. Serious sunbathing will be out for at least six months after a course of treatment, and a sun block should be applied to the skin whenever there is any danger of it being exposed to the sun's harmful rays.

To deal with an area of pigmentation, several treatment sessions may be required at intervals of between six to twelve weeks, although superficial pigmented lesions can often be cleared after two to four sessions.

## Results

Although it is possible to remove many superficial skin disorders permanently in the areas treated, in some cases only a partial lightening will occur. For this reason it is wise to seek an opinion from several reputable surgeons in order to gain a more accurate assessment of your own individual problem and how well laser treatment is likely to work for you.

## Potential Complications

At the hands of a reputable and experienced surgeon, the chances of any complications arising are pretty rare.

## Liposuction

Sometimes referred to as lipolysis or suction lipectomy, liposuction should not be viewed as a cure for obesity, nor an instant slimming method for the lazy. In cases, however, where dieting and exercise have failed to reduce localised areas of stubborn spot fat it can be a useful means of effecting the final alterations or refinements to body size or shape that often elude many successful slimmers. Most surgeons will not operate on those who still need to shed a good proportion of superfluous fat, and even when this has been achieved, they prefer to wait until the prospective patient's weight has been stabilised for a period of months.

Liposuction works best on traditionally difficult-to-lose fat deposits that accumulate (as a result of hereditary factors) in areas such as the hips, thighs, buttocks, abdomen, arms and waist. Saddle-bag thighs, fat knees, pot bellies, double chins, spare tyres, 'love-handles' and underarm deposits are all areas that are said to respond well to this type of cosmetic procedure.

## Penile Implants

Impotence is a word with which few men feel comfortable. The merest prospect of it happening to them is enough to stir up all kinds of deeply buried fears, emotions and insecurities. The fact is, however, that most men are likely to suffer from it at some point or another in their lives. In most cases, the cause and the cure is likely to be within the sufferer's own control. If certain contributory factors – such as alcohol consumption, pressure of work, financial or family worries and stress – are allowed to become a problem, they can all affect a man's ability to attain and/or maintain an erection. Remove the cause and, in the majority of cases, the cure will take care of itself.

Occasionally, a single incident of impotence can trigger off a self-perpetuating cycle of anxiety that grows with each repeated failure until the fear of failure itself becomes a self-fulfilling prophecy. In many cases, some form of therapy or counselling is often all that is required to help men suffering from this problem to break their pattern of anxiety, regain their perspective, and return their lives to normal.

In a small minority of cases, the sexual dysfunction will have an organic cause – the man may, for example, be suffering from diabetes, vascular disease or some other physiological problem that is affecting his ability to attain erection. In such cases, a penile implant may be the only solution.

Inserting a penile implant is a specialised procedure best carried out by a urologist rather than a cosmetic surgeon. There are currently two main types of implant available. The first predominantly consists of two silicone rods. Depending on the type chosen, these will either be fairly rigid (in which case the patient may have to learn to cope with the embarrassing experience of appearing to have a permanent erection), or flexible enough to enable the penis to be bent. The second type consists of a silicone rubber balloon which can be inflated at will by means of a special reservoir and pump. When an erection is required, the man simply pumps a valve which allows the fluid to enter the penis. When the valve is released, the fluid returns to the reservoir.

In both instances the surgical procedure, which takes approximately two hours, is carried out under general anaesthetic.

If the silicone rods are used, these will be inserted straight into the penile shaft. With the inflatable device, the surgeon will make an incision in the lower abdomen, just above the root of the penis, into which he will then insert two inflatable tubes attached to a fluid-filled reservoir which, in turn, is connected to a pump secreted in the scrotum.

There may be considerable swelling around the genitals plus a fair degree of pain and discomfort which may last for several months. Providing there are no complications, most patients should be able to return to work after two weeks' convalescence, but sexual intercourse will be banned for at least another four, and in some cases six, weeks.

### Hospitalisation Period
Seven to ten days.

### Potential Complications
These include all the usual risks of infection that accompany any form of surgery, as well as persistent pain or discomfort. With the inflatable type of implant there is an added risk of fluid leaking from the reservoir.

In Britain, suitable patients can have this operation free of charge on the National Health Service. As government-funded health facilities elsewhere are likely to vary, patients residing outside Britain should seek the advice of their doctor.


# CYTOTOXIC FOOD-ALLERGY TESTING (AND OBESITY)

Over the years, a number of popular hypotheses have been proposed that supposedly provide a rational explanation for the sudden development of, and subsequent inability to lose, surplus fat. One of the most popular, and most widely believed, is the theory that fat is a simple calorific equation – if you take in more calories than your body can burn up, the surplus energy will be stored as fat. The only truly effective solution, we are told, is to restrict the number of calories we ingest daily in the form of food. When fewer calories are consumed than are required to keep the body functioning, the body's miraculous ability to make up any deficit automatically causes stored fat to be released from its fat cells.

This sounds perfectly logical in theory, and in practice it often works to most people's satisfaction. But, as many overweight people will testify, there are several flaws in this hypothesis. For a significant number of people, dieting – restricting calorie intake – is largely ineffective at providing a permanent solution to their weight problems.

A second theory that has gained much credence relates to the rate at which each individual's metabolism works. If you are lucky enough to have a high metabolic rate, your body will be so efficient at burning up calories that you will be able to eat as much as you like, and still not gain any excess weight. Conversely, those with a low metabolic rate may well find that even a restricted number of calories could cause them to gain weight.

A third theory is that what matters is not so much what you eat, or how much, but the time of day at which you eat it, and the way you combine the different food groups. According to this theory, mixing alkaline-producing foods and those that produce acid at the same meal can create an adverse effect on the digestive process, which in turn can lead to poor assimilation of nutrients, inefficient digestion and subsequent weight problems.

The fact is, there are as many different theories that purport to provide a 'definitive' explanation as to why we put on weight as there are foods that supposedly make us fat. But by far the best, the most helpful and the most logical hypothesis I have come across in over 20 years of research into dieting and health is one that is gaining more and more credence with each new piece of research – that the majority of people who have an inexplicable resistance to most dieting and weight-loss regimes are simply suffering from a masked allergy or sensitivity to one or more items of food that they habitually eat. In my opinion, this theory not only makes enormous sense, but it also provides a perfectly feasible explanation as to why some people cannot lose weight no matter how much they restrict their calorie intake, and why others who have succeeded in losing several pounds after weeks of stringent dieting, often regain virtually all of their lost weight after just one small binge.

Cytotoxic testing was originally established to service the needs of the medical profession and police investigations. It has been used successfully in the United States, Australia, New Zealand and Scandinavia for over 30 years to treat an extensive range of physiological and behavioural problems including asthma, eczema, migraine, obesity, digestive disorders, rheumatism and hyperactivity. It is a scientifically proven method of identifying with at least 80-per-cent accuracy, a wide range of foodstuffs and environmental agents to which you may be either allergic, intolerant or sensitive.

One surprising side-effect of cytotoxic testing has slowly emerged. After identifying and eliminating the specific foods that were pinpointed as causing their allergic reactions, many people have been delighted also to discover that they had shed several pounds in weight. Further trials and studies have revealed that there does indeed appear to be an important connection between food sensitivity and sudden weight gains, as well as a persistent resistance to 'normal' methods of weight loss.

Cytotoxic tests can be carried out in one of two ways. Some organisations such as the York Nutritional Laboratory in England prefer to work in association with their client's doctor. Others, such as Larkhall Natural Health, based in London, will work directly with the client. In the case of the former, clients first have to liaise with their own doctor, arrange for their test to be booked with York and then get their doctor to take the blood sample according to specific instructions issued by the laboratory. The blood sample should be taken as late in the day as possible, after a 12-hour fast, and it should be mailed to the laboratory the same evening to enable the tests to be carried out within 24 hours.

If the latter course is chosen using an organisation such as Larkhall, the client books the test in advance, the blood is taken during a visit to the company's premises by specially trained personnel and the tests are conducted within six hours. According to Dr Robert Woodward of Larkhall, a test carried out within six hours of taking the blood sample is likely to be far more accurate than a test carried out on blood that is 24 hours old.

Both tests are performed using a small sample (around 10 ml) of blood from which the leucocytes (white blood cells) are removed. Suspensions of the leucocytes are then mixed with extracts of each food to be tested. After a period of incubation, the suspensions are examined by microscope to assess the extent to which the leucocytes may have reacted against any of the extracts.

In simple terms, those foods which the body recognises as an 'invader' (such as those that cause the allergic reaction) will be surrounded and attacked by defender cells called neutrophils in an attempt to phagocytose or 'eat' them. This phagocytic activity results in a number of vacuoles or 'bubbles' being created inside the neutrophil. Assessing the number of bubbles enables the analyst to determine the severity of the reaction to the particular food involved.

### Benefits and Claims

According to Mr M. Varey, one of the proprietors and chief analysts at the York Nutritional Laboratory (and also many other experts who have conducted intensive research into this field), you only need to be 'sensitive' to a specific food or ingredient to experience an almost instant allergic reaction which can, and often does, result in retaining an excessive amount of water. The difference between a food allergy and a food sensitivity is that the former is fixed, and therefore likely to remain with you for life, while the latter, sometimes referred to as a cyclic allergy, can often be cured by avoiding the foods that are known to trigger a reaction for two to three months. A food sensitivity can cause puffiness around the eyes, swellings in the neck and ankles, abdominal distension and a collection of fluid in the fatty tissue surrounding the hips and thighs – in other words, all the areas where women are especially prone to accumulating and storing fat.

Because science has not yet been able to determine precisely *how* such a reaction is triggered, the only currently known method for controlling this widespread problem is through the identification and avoidance of all those foods to which one is known to be sensitive. After a period of total elimination, some people may never experience a return of their original symptoms. Others may not be so fortunate insofar as their symptoms may recur several months later when their original sensitivity has had time to rebuild itself.

There is another problem – probably more widespread than many weight-prone people suspect – with the way in which many food sensitivities often work. It seems that they cause us to develop a craving for and addiction to the very foods to which we are most intolerant. This makes it all the more difficult for us to give them up. According to Mr Varey, eating a food to which you are sensitive sets off a chain reaction within the body, and the more you eat this food, the more severe the reaction becomes. Food sensitivities are believed to challenge and weaken the immune system. When this occurs, the digestive process suffers, which in turn results in undigested protein matter being absorbed into the bloodstream. The body's defence mechanism then comes into play with the result that, having identified the undigested matter as a foreign invader, the system then acts to encapsulate it in a fat cell and flood it with water to dilute the effect.

With a cytotoxic food-allergy test it is now possible not only to determine potential allergic reactions to a vast array of foodstuffs and ingredients, but also the severity of the reaction. For example, a typical test result may reveal a relatively mild (classified as a 'group 1') sensitivity to dairy products, which means that you can continue to eat these foods normally; a moderate (or 'group 2') sensitivity to wheat and grains, which means that these should be restricted or rotated; and a severe ('group 3') intolerance to yeast, coffee, chocolate and certain fruits, in which case you would be advised to avoid these particular foods altogether for a few months. To complicate matters even further, abstaining from any group 3 sensitive foods will undoubtedly cause you to experience some initial withdrawal symptoms.

## Results

Apart from appearing to be of enormous benefit in identifying specific foods that can trigger an attack of asthma and migraine, eczema flare-ups, hyperactivity in children, and a number of other allergic reactions, cytotoxic food-allergy testing may well prove to offer a definitive solution to the prayers of many people who, based on the amount of food they actually eat, really do not deserve to have a persistent problem with their weight.

Although the British medical profession *per se* remains somewhat sceptical still about cytotoxic testing, especially in relation to weight, a number of studies and trials have revealed that impressive results have been achieved by a number of people, simply by eliminating those foods to which they have been shown to have a sensitivity. However, as we have already discovered with cellulite, there is no such thing as an overnight cure (although something approaching it has been achieved by a few people who have managed to shed as much as 14 pounds in as little as 7 days). If you really are determined to solve your weight problems once and for all, and a food sensitivity has been identified as a potential – though not necessarily a guaranteed – cause of your problem, you will have to dedicate yourself to making some possibly drastic and certainly long-term alterations to your diet.

## Value for Money?

It is a known fact that more and more people are developing a sensitivity or reaction to a variety of different allergenic substances, including food. Whether this is a direct result of the agricultural and food industry's increasing reliance on the

---

**AVERAGE PRICE**

Costs vary according to the number of foods you wish to be included in the test. As a rule of thumb, a standard test which includes between 80–100 of the most common allergy-causing foods will cost approximately ۩ ۩ ۩ ۩ ۩

use of chemicals, pesticides, additives and preservatives, or whether it is due to a combination of potentially toxic environmental factors remains yet to be proven to the scientist's conclusive satisfaction. Meanwhile, however, the fact remains that the incidence of food and environment-related allergic reactions has risen sharply in recent years. Apart from the yet-to-be proven weight problems this may potentially cause, the implications on our overall health and well-being are unmistakably clear.

For this reason, I am inclined to believe that cytotoxic food-allergy testing represents reasonable value for money. Although the amount of money involved is actually quite high, it works out favourably when compared to the amount the average overweight person is likely to spend during the course of a year on other weight-loss methods. Therefore, if you are desperate for a solution to your weight problems, and all other methods and/or serious attempts at shedding weight have failed, a cytotoxic test is definitely worth considering. It could even prove to be worth saving up for, especially if experience has taught you that one small binge after weeks of dieting can result in an inexplicable overnight gain of several pounds.

# DEPILATION

When it comes to hair-removal, most women prefer to do this for themselves in the comfort of their own homes. Although using a depilatory cream is undeniably cheaper than visiting a salon, and probably much more convenient, most salon-based depilation treatments have two advantages: firstly, they are likely to be more efficient at removing unwanted hair; and secondly, any regrowth takes much longer to appear.

## *Propil Hair-growth Inhibitor*

Propil (which stands for 'progressive and lasting depilation') is a special hair-growth retardant treatment unique to the

French cosmetic brand G.M. Collin. Available in certain salons throughout Britain and Europe, Propil is becoming a popular add-on treatment to waxing.

The active ingredient in Propil is papine, an extract of papaya which destroys the hair germ cells through its enzyme action. The whole process is carried out in a tight sequence which involves waxing a small area with a 'non-residue' type wax, then stippling on the Propil gel immediately afterwards using a stiff brush. The process is repeated over and over again until the entire area has been waxed and treated.

As with electrolysis, it is important to carry out a thorough consultation first in order to determine the course of hair growth. Appointments must be timed carefully at intervals of two to four weeks, and then spaced in accordance with the reduction in growth procedure.

### Benefits and Claims

This therapy results in a significant reduction in hair growth. It can safely be used on the face and the body, and is claimed to be a painless and extremely effective alternative to electrolysis.

### Results

Because Propil inhibits hair growth by gradually causing the germ cell to atrophy and die, it may take anything from 15–20 sessions to become and remain completely free of superfluous hair. Meanwhile, any regrowth is likely to be patchy and uneven.

If by the sixth session you have not noticed a marked reduction in hair growth, you should discontinue the treatment. Although this is not particularly common, there are certain individual physiological factors, and one or two drugs (such as cortisone and some forms of hormone) that can have an adverse influence on the action of the gel.

---

**AVERAGE PRICE**

**♉**

(plus cost of waxing)

---

### Value for Money?

If you have your legs waxed regularly, and you can find a local salon that offers this treatment, this is priced keenly enough to be worth adding on to your normal treatment as an experiment. If it works — and there are plenty who say it does — the extra initial expense could save you a fortune in waxing later on.

## Sugaring

Based on a technique that has been practised in the Middle East for thousands of years, sugaring is currently enjoying something of a revival as a reasonably cheap alternative to waxing. A thick, viscous solution made from sugar, lemon, herbs and water is warmed and then massaged onto the skin. As the solution cools it hardens just enough to enable the therapist to grip the glutinous toffee-like edges and, with a quick, sharp flick of the wrist, rip it away in sections from the skin taking the hair beneath with it. It is slightly messier than using wax, but, if it is done correctly and efficiently, it should also be marginally less painful. Your skin may be red and slightly sensitive for a few hours after treatment.

### Benefits and Claims
When hair is removed from the roots, any regrowth will take longer to appear.

### Results
Effects last 4–6 weeks. If the therapist is not sufficiently experienced at applying and removing the substance, certain areas may require more than one attempt. People with sensitive skin should try a patch test first. If waxing makes your skin react, or seems to encourage ingrowing hairs, the chances are that sugaring probably will too.

### Value for Money?
Debatable, but if you can find a therapist who is skilful and adept it is worth experimenting with.

---

**AVERAGE PRICE**

ʊ

## Waxing

A thin, glutinous layer of hot wax is applied to the skin. A thicker, denser variety of wax is used for the bikini-line area. The wax is ripped off when it has reached a certain stage of dryness.

### Benefits and Claims

Removes hair from the roots, and has an inhibiting effect on regrowth, which can take up to six weeks to appear.

### Results

Effective but very painful. Some people find that repeated waxing gradually weakens the hair until it becomes finer and thinner, and may even disappear altogether in some areas.

### Value for Money?

If you have a high pain threshold, low skin-sensitivity, and do not mind displaying furry legs for a few weeks in between appointments (to be effective, waxing is best done on hair that is a minimum of a quarter of an inch in length), then you might regard this as good value for money. Otherwise, stick to a razor.

| AVERAGE PRICE |
| :---: |
| ʊ ʊ |

## FACIAL MASKS

Every year the beauty industry invests billions of dollars of its vast profits in researching and developing new products, and inventing ingenious new methods for making their existing products work more efficiently. One of the latest innovations to capture the imagination of salon owners and clients alike is the facial mask.

Until recently, facial masks usually consisted of thick, spread-on-wash-off creams, muds or clays, whose sole purpose was to deep-cleanse the skin of impurities and prepare it for the main facial treatment that followed. The tendency today, however, is to employ a scientifically formulated range of materials which have been specially designed to form or set into a mask-like structure that is itself the treatment.

As virtually every major cosmetic house or manufacturer has devised and launched its own facial-mask treatment, testing and reviewing the merits of each one would not only have taken up far too much valuable research time, but would also fill far more space than is reasonable in this guide. I have therefore confined the information in this section to a brief overview of the more popular types of facial masks that are currently finding favour with a large number of salon-owners and their clients.

## Collagen Masks

Collagen is a protein substance that binds together all the cells in the body. An important constituent in healthy bone, cartilage and the dermis, collagen and elastin fibres are responsible for the toughness and elasticity of all the structures supported by the body's connective tissue. As we age, the amount of collagen in the skin begins to deteriorate. This leads to progressive dehydration, loss of elasticity and an overall weakening in the tissue causing the skin to sag and fine lines and wrinkles to appear. The use of collagen as a beauty aid is a fairly recent innovation. Prior to this it had mainly been used by French surgeons who had found it helpful in repairing and healing wounds and burns.

A typical collagen-mask treatment will commence with a preparatory deep-cleansing and gentle skin-peeling routine. This will be followed by the application of a special serum designed to nourish and hydrate the skin. Next, a paper-thin sheet of collagen (usually prepared from the muscle fibre of young cattle) will be taken from a sterile pack and placed over the face and neck. Slits will be made in the sheet to accommodate the nose, and to enable it to be shaped to fit the neck. A special collagen-containing lotion will then be sprayed or sponged on to the mask in order to hydrate it and ensure it adheres to the skin. The mask will then be rehydrated every ten minutes or so until the treatment is complete.

At the end of the session, which usually takes an hour and a quarter, the mask is detached from the skin by first rolling a section around a tissue, and then rolling the tissue upwards from the neck. The skin is then moisturised with a special cream or lotion specifically designed to support and enhance the collagen treatment.

### Benefits and Claims
The strength of the claims made for collagen-mask treatments will vary from salon to salon. These can range from the spectacular, such as those that promise to turn back the years by 'inducing intensive cellular regeneration', to the less fanciful and slightly more realistic ones, such as those that focus on providing 'strength and support to existing fibres in order to help slow down the rate of degeneration'.

### Results
Collagen masks certainly give the complexion a boost, providing a soft, smooth, glowing effect that lasts for several days. But if you are looking for a miracle cure, this is not it. If, on the other hand, you merely wish to make the most of your skin, to help preserve what you have got for as long as possible and to prevent further deterioration, regular collagen-mask treatments can prove to be a marvellous aid.

### Warning
Reactions to collagen masks are pretty rare, but if you are allergic to certain foods, especially meat, it might be wise to ask if you can have a patch test first.

### Value for Money?
On the basis that results are supposed to be progressive, and the best results are said to be achieved when a course of five weekly treatments is taken, this could prove to be a rather expensive beauty preservation experiment. It might, however,

---

**AVERAGE PRICE**

From

ʊʊʊʊ

be worth investing in occasionally, perhaps as a once or twice-yearly maintenance treatment.

## Modelling Masks

A 'modelling-mask' facial involves an application of a special paste that moulds itself around the contours of the face as it dries. Once dry, it forms into a thick, one-piece layer of rubbery material, rather like the latex moulds children use to make model figures – hence its name.

Most modelling-mask treatments take about one hour to complete. The first stage usually consists of a preparation treatment to cleanse the skin thoroughly, followed by the application and removal of a gentle peeling cream to remove any dead or dry surface skin cells. Any comedones (blackheads) will then be extracted prior to the application of specific plant or marine-based oils or creams which are massaged into the skin, either manually or with the aid of a galvanic current. Finally, the ingredients of the modelling mask are mixed together and pasted on to the neck and face with a spatula in an even layer (avoiding the eyes, nostrils and mouth) and left for 15–20 minutes to dry. As it dries the mask heats up to a pleasurable temperature (usually around 42°C). This helps open the pores so that the nutrients contained in the creams can be better absorbed. Once dry, the modelling mask is peeled off in a single layer, the face is cleansed and a final layer of moisturising cream or lotion specifically selected to suit your individual skin type or problem is applied.

### Benefits and Claims

Modelling masks are said to be suitable for all skin types. Their primary value is said to lie in the fact that they help increase the penetration of active ingredients, stimulate cutaneous function, and hydrate and tone the skin.

### Results

While they certainly appear to make an immediate difference

to the tone, texture and appearance of facial skin, it is difficult to assess whether these masks are actually any more effective or beneficial than many other types of facial treatments.

## Value for Money?

Unless you are claustrophobic, you will probably find the experience extremely pleasurable and relaxing. Treatment is recommended once or twice monthly. A monthly treatment should be enough for most people with a fairly normal skin, and on that basis it is certainly good value for money.

# GUINOT CATHIODERMIE

Developed 35 years ago by French cosmetic chemist René Guinot, Cathiodermie (which is marketed under the name of Hydradermie in continental Europe and the United States) first became available in Britain in the early 1980s. Since then it has rapidly become one of the most respected, and consequently one of the most popular, forms of facial treatment available today.

A session of Guinot Cathiodermie should last between 60 and 90 minutes, depending upon the specific treatment you are having. The majority of treatments incorporate the use of a mild and totally painless electrical galvanic current in conjunction with different extracts of herbs, fruits, flowers and sea plants in gel form to improve the skin texture and treat difficult skin problems such as acne.

After superficially cleansing the skin of make-up, surface grime and oiliness, the therapist will apply a special solution called Electro Z, designed to help speed up the skin's metabolism and reduce its resistance to the mild galvanic current. Having selected a specific plant-extract gel suitable for your skin type, the therapist will then massage this into the skin with the aid of two fine stainless steel rollers which emit the galvanic current. Although this process sounds frightening, it is quite pain-free and relaxing. The galvanic current draws the ionised gel into the pores where it gets to work dissolving impurities and any accumulated sebum.

Next comes the extraction process. Although not as painful as extracting teeth, some people might find this part of the treatment a mite uncomfortable physically, as well as quite embarrassing psychologically. (To my mind, having someone peering closely into your pores through a magnifying glass and triumphantly exclaiming 'Ah ha!' whenever she spies an errant blackhead lurking within, is somewhat akin to the embarrassing experience of having your mother-in-law notice the existence of your prized cobweb collection!) Nonetheless, extraction is a vital part of a Cathiodermie treatment, and once this part is over, you will, no doubt, be pleased to have a clear complexion.

This is followed by the application of a special oxygenated emulsion ($OZ^2$) on top of which is placed a piece of fine gauze. On goes the machine again, and this time a perspex rod with a bulb on the end will be passed over the face for several minutes. The high-frequency current passing through the bulb will bathe the skin in a sterilising anti-bacterial, germicidal ozone, healing imperfections and drying up spots as it goes.

The final steps consist of a relaxing massage with a special nourishing fluid (Relax Gel Lifting), followed by a Geloide Prescription Mask, and the application of a moisturiser specially selected to suit your individual skin type.

There are six different types of Guinot Cathiodermie treatments available, each designed to treat a specific area. While all are basically similar in terms of gel extracts, massage technique and the use of galvanic and/or high-frequency current, they differ slightly depending upon which area of the body is being treated. All Cathiodermie treatments are designed to help normalise your skin's pH balance and stimulate cellular metabolism.

## Eye Cathiodermie

Often recommended as a two-stage treatment with a three-day interval between each phase, Eye Cathiodermie is marketed as a both a remedial and preventive treatment for the delicate area around the eye. Three special ingredients essential to the skin's elasticity – elastin, collagen and mucopolysaccharides – are used to reduce fine lines, shadows, puffiness, bags, crow's feet and wrinkles.

## Neck Cathiodermie

Another two-stage treatment (though some salons dispense with the second stage), neck cathiodermie specialises in helping to combat and correct the gradual progression of ageing lines and wrinkles in the neck and throat area.

## Back Cathiodermie

A two-stage treatment with a course of four to six sessions recommended for best results, Back Cathiodermie concentrates on treating spotty or acne-prone backs and generally improving the texture of the skin in this often neglected area. This is achieved through exfoliation with a body scrub and the application of specific gel extracts. As this treatment also incorporates massage of the back, neck and shoulders, it is said to be excellent for easing strain away from tense muscles. For this reason, Back Cathiodermie is suitable for, and popular with, both sexes.

## Bust Cathiodermie

This treatment is purported to revitalise and tone the network of underlying connective tissue that supports the breasts, resulting in firmer, more youthful breasts. For best results, a course of two treatments per week over three to four weeks is recommended.

## Super-Cathiodermie

This superior 90-minute treatment combines all the techniques used in Eye, Neck and Face Cathiodermie. Super-Cathiodermie uses formulations containing a high concentration of active principles aimed specifically at treating and solving the problems associated with ageing in these areas. For those who are ultra-conscious of their face and body, it is suggested that Super-Cathiodermie should be alternated with a monthly Cathiodermie Facial treatment.

## Bio-Peeling

A one-hour treatment involving the gentle removal of every trace of dry surface skin. This treatment is said to leave a beautiful matt complexion of firm young cells. Recommended for oily, congested and teenage skins.

### Results

A superior form of treatment in every way. The massage element is immensely relaxing, the products are exquisite and the treatment is decidedly beneficial. Not only did my tester's skin glow for weeks afterwards, but she declared Cathiodermie to be the best, most relaxing and beneficial of all the facial treatments she sampled throughout the entire course of her research for this book. In fact, she was so impressed with the results, she is even considering making a regular monthly appointment. Coming from someone who has always held a strong aversion to any form of 'hands-on' treatment, this is praise indeed!

### Bonus

To safeguard their reputation and the quality of their treatments, René Guinot insist that all qualified beauty therapists attend a four-day training session at their own headquarters before they will allow any salon to purchase their equipment or offer any Cathiodermie treatments. This ensures that all

Cathiodermie therapists receive a standardised training (after which they are subjected to stringent testing procedures before being awarded the Guinot certificate) and, therefore, the techniques used should always be the same whether you are visiting a salon in this country or in any other part of the world.

## Warning
Because of the electrical galvanic and high-frequency currents used in Cathiodermie treatments, there are certain circumstances in which this form of treatment is not advised:

- If you have metal plates or a pacemaker fitted.
- If you are epileptic.
- If you are pregnant (although the treatment is perfectly safe, you might feel awkward or uncomfortable lying still for such a long time).
- Immediately prior to a special event (as all the impurities are brought to the surface, your skin could become spotty a few days afterwards. For this reason it is best to book your treatment at least seven days in advance).
- Within four hours of any form of heat treatment (such as a sauna, jacuzzi or sunbed), or facial waxing.
- Immediately following electrolysis or any other form of electrical treatment.

Clients are also advised not to apply any make-up other than lipstick for at least six hours after a Cathiodermie facial.

## Value for Money?
As Cathiodermie treatments really do seem to have a beneficial effect on the skin, and they are not overly expensive, a facial once every four to six weeks is terrific value for money. Courses of treatment taken over a shorter period of time could, however, create quite a burden on your bank account. On the other hand, if you are seriously seeking a solution to a specific, long-standing skin problem, this undoubtedly ranks as a treatment well worth trying.

---

**AVERAGE PRICE**

**Facial Cathiodermie**
**ŲŲ**

**Eye Cathiodermie:**
Day 1 **ŲŲ**
Day 4 **ŲŲ**

**Neck Cathiodermie:**
Day 1 **ŲŲ**
Day 4 **ŲŲ**

**Back Cathiodermie:**
Day 1 **ŲŲŲ**
Day 4 **ŲŲ**

**Bust Cathiodermie**
**(many salons offer price reductions when a course of treatments is booked)**
**Super Cathiodermie**
**ŲŲŲ**

**Bio-Peeling**
**ŲŲ**

# HAIR-LOSS TREATMENTS

If there is one aspect of our appearance that is likely to cause equal concern to men and women alike it is the state, quantity and condition of the hair on our heads. Taken for granted in our youth, alternately abused or neglected according to each fickle phase of fashion that influences our teenage years, our hair is rarely given sufficient attention, or even the appreciation it deserves, until we are jolted by the realisation that it is impossible to retrieve what we have already lost.

Going grey and going bald are our two major hair concerns. Women worry about the former, and men have a horror of the latter. But neither sex gets much sympathy from the other when their fears are expressed. Men fear balding because they think it makes them look old and less attractive. Women fear going grey for precisely the same reasons. But few women can relate to men's fears because their perception of male attractiveness very often has little to do with a man's looks or his age. And the reason men cannot relate to women's fear of going grey is because, to them, this is infinitely preferable to going bald.

There are far more solutions to greyness than there are to baldness. And because baldness is predominantly a male problem (although it can occur in women, especially after the menopause), this is one area of their appearance which can make men every bit as susceptible to 'miracle baldness cures' as women are to 'magical slimming remedies'. In order to understand what can and cannot be achieved in terms of restoring hair or slowing down hair loss, it is necessary first to know something about the process of hair growth and the conditions that affect it.

Every hair has its own life cycle: firstly, it is 'born'; then it has a six-month period of growth followed by a three-month rest period, at the end of which it dies and falls out to be replaced by another hair. On average, each hair grows about half an inch every month during the growth period, and shedding takes place during the resting phase at the rate of between

30–150 hairs per day. The average head of hair contains 100,000 or so hairs, of which 85 per cent will be in the growing phase, and the remaining 15 per cent in a resting phase, at any one time.

One of the primary causes of poor hair growth, excessive hair loss and thinning is a deficiency of nutrients reaching the scalp to nourish the hair follicles. Severe dieting, illness, toxins, drugs, poor nutrition, stress, overwork, hormonal fluctuations, trauma and even childbirth can all disturb the body's essential ecological pattern, altering the metabolic process and depriving the cells of the vital nutrients required for the promotion of healthy hair growth. And because the external pressures of work, finances, and the daily stresses of life are mounting, women are just as likely to seek help for a severe hair problem these days as men.

The other major cause of hair loss is a genetically inherited biological mechanism that predisposes certain individuals to develop androgenic alopecia, more commonly known as male pattern baldness (MPB). The symptoms of MPB are easily recognisable, and will often manifest during puberty. These include an excessively greasy scalp and an unusual amount of hairs being shed each time the hair is washed.

It has long been rumoured that bald men are more virile than their hirsute brothers. This common supposition, which may indeed have some basis in fact, arose out of the discovery that the male hormones androgen and testosterone have long been known to be linked to MPB (androgen is responsible for the male physical characteristics, and testosterone governs the sex drive). For some time it was thought that reducing the amount of male hormones with oestrogen treatment could counteract androgenic hair loss. This practice was soon dropped when it was found that it could cause the embarrassing development of female characteristics. Applied topically to the scalp, however, oestrogen is not only quite safe, but can also be quite effective in arresting the symptoms of MPB.

More recent research seems to indicate that, while the male

hormones do have a part to play in MPB, they are not the whole of the story. According to the research conducted by one company, La Biosthetique, which specialises in treating hair disorders, MPB occurs when an abnormal genetic coding allows a specific enzyme, 5 Alpha Reductase, to penetrate the cell. 'Once inside it transforms the male hormone testosterone into dehydrotestosterone which has the power of over-stimu-lating the cellular metabolism. The sebaceous glands will produce excessive sebum (which makes the hair greasy) and the hair cell's metabolic rate is increased giving it a shorter life span. The life cycle is therefore reduced and the follicle quickly exhausts its capability to produce new hair.'

Fortunately, many hair problems that have traditionally been difficult to treat are now finding successful cures through new methods of treatment, such as massage, ultraviolet and infra–red light or electrical stimulation. Expensive drugs such as Minoxidil, and the more recently-developed Tricomin (which is currently undergoing trials in France), are appar-ently offering astonishing results in certain cases. And it has now been discovered that even those with a genetic predis-position towards MPB can do much to halt or prevent any further loss of hair if they start preventive treatment early enough. But as some of these therapies and treatments are still in the experimental stages, the following information is confined to reviewing only the most widely available options.

## Hair Transplants

Developed in the 1950s by an American surgeon, this proce-dure involves transplanting hair follicles from the back and/or either side of the head (where the hair generally lasts the longest) to the crown and/or temples. Performed under local anaesthetic, several sessions may be required (at minimum intervals of at least one month) to remove a series of grafts of hair-growing skin from the donor site and implant these at the recipient site on top of the head. Each session is likely to take around four to five hours, and great skill is required to ensure that the transplanted plugs of hair grow in the correct direction.

After treatment, a turban-like bandage will be applied to the head to cover both sites, and you will be given some form of cap to wear over this for anything up to 48 hours. You will be banned from washing your hair for at least five to seven days, and from touching the recipient site for several more days after that. You may feel a little discomfort initially as small crusts form and dry over each graft, but these usually fall off some time around the third week. Any resulting scars should be hidden once the transplants begin to produce hair.

### Benefits and Claims

Although it takes approximately three months for the hair to grow through, any new growth should be permanent. However, if any later hair loss should occur in the region of the original donor site at the sides or back of the head, the transplanted follicles will inevitably suffer too.

### Results

Best results are usually achieved with Caucasian hair. In most cases, this is likely to be successful and relatively permanent. It is important, however, to remember that hair transplants do not create *new* hair, they merely redistribute what you already have. Consequently, no amount of transplants can re-create the appearance of an abundant mop of hair. What you are more likely to end up with is a greater covering of hair that may look as if it is thinning.

The only complication that tends to arise is the occasional failure of a graft to 'take'. But providing you choose a reputable clinic or surgeon, it is a fairly normal practice for these to be replaced without charge.

### Value for Money?

Yes – if your confidence is directly related to the volume of hair on your head.

---

**AVERAGE PRICE**

Variable but likely to be quite expensive (you could probably fly Concorde across the Atlantic for less).

## Warning Note

Patients with heart problems and those taking anti-coagulant drugs need to advise their surgeon of their condition, as the local anaesthetics used in this procedure usually contain vaso-constrictors which have the contradictory effect of making the blood coagulate.

## La Biosthetique

Established in 1946 by French biologist, writer and humanist Marcel Contier, La Biosthetique operates a service that is broadly similar to that offered by the Lazartigue organisation (see page 87). Instead of owning their own advisory centres, however, La Biosthetique claim to be a less commercial and more specialised organisation whose service is available only through a selected number of salons worldwide.

Salons operating this scheme usually (though not always) offer a free consultation and analysis service. This involves filling in a detailed questionnaire and extracting samples of hair from your head, both of which are then sent off to La Biosthetique to be examined and analysed. The diagnosis and recommended programme of treatment are returned to the salon within seven to fourteen days, at which time you will be given comprehensive instructions on how to use each product prescribed to help treat your specific problem.

## Benefits and Claims

La Biosthetique products are said to be able to treat a number of 'problem hair' and hair-loss conditions. These include andro-genic alopecia; alopecia aerata; hyperhydrosis (an excessive scalp perspiration condition which, when associated with stress or over-work, can dramatically affect hair quality and quantity); scalp induration (tightening of the scalp); and chemotherapy-induced hair loss. All preparations are claimed to originate solely from natural sources.

## Results

Difficult to verify. According to Biosthetique's impressive explanatory document on hair loss, however, the following results are claimed to be obtainable with regular use of the preparations prescribed (the document not only gives a clear description and analysis of the cause of each hair problem, but also provides a detailed explanation of why and how each prescribed treatment works):

- Androgenic alopecia – can be slowed down to between 30–80 per cent, and in some cases completely controlled.
- Alopecia aerata – hair normally grows back within one to three months. Unfortunately, in many cases the new hair grows back completely white.
- Hyperhydrosis – beneficial results are quickly noticeable.
- Scalp induration – no results given, but this condition is claimed to be 'not difficult to treat'.
- Chemotherapy-induced hair loss – the results of on-going trials conducted in collaboration with doctors and hospitals in Scotland, England and Eire have so far been declared a resounding success. Every case treated was expected to incur total hair loss, but in the worst case to date only 30 per cent of the hair was lost. In two specific cases where repeated chemotherapy treatment had resulted in total hair loss, the hair of both patients began to regrow within three to four weeks of commencing treatment with La Biosthetique products and continued to grow despite further chemotherapy sessions.

---

**AVERAGE PRICE**

Depends on the number of products prescribed and duration of treatment. As a rule of thumb, one month's supply of the cheapest product – a shampoo – costs on average ᙏ but in cases of male pattern baldness, lifetime treatment may be required.

---

## Value for Money?

Based on the results claimed (and it is hard to envisage a company of this size making exaggerated claims, or conducting hospital trials that cannot be substantiated), this could be good value for money. As always, however, it is advisable to obtain detailed information on the true costs involved, and the potential for success, before committing yourself to treatment.

## *J.F. Lazartigue Diagnostic & Advisory Hair Centre*

With over 125 advisory centres spread throughout 25 countries, Jean-Francois Lazartigue's empire is not to be confused
with a chain of up-market hair salons. These specialist centres'
sole *raison d'être* is founded upon diagnosing and devising the
ultimate solution to problem hair.

The consultation service is free. With the aid of a small,
powerful microscope, a specially trained therapist will look
closely at the state of the root and shaft of your hair, and
analyse your scalp to identify any weaknesses or problems of
hair condition or structure. Having diagnosed the cause of your
difficulties, she will then devise a personal programme of hair
and scalp treatment based on Lazartigue products to be used
at home. Some problems, such as alopecia aerata (a hair-loss
disorder connected with stress, overwork and certain other
nervous conditions), may require a three-month intensive
course of treatment; others, such as MPB, may require a longer
(in some cases indefinite) period of treatment in order to maintain any slow-down achieved in the rate of hair loss. Any
further check-ups (recommended at three-monthly intervals)
are also free of charge.

### *Benefits and Claims*
Lazartigue's hair-care products are claimed to be preventive
and curative.

### *Results*
Impossible to predict. Although Lazartigue profess to be able
to address and cure many hair problems, and to halt others,
it is very difficult to obtain any definitive evidence or proof.

### *Value for Money?*
Impossible to assess in the absence of any real proof. If the
sheer number of their centres is anything to go by, Lazartigue
must be doing something right. Even so, it would be worth
investigating what supportive evidence they can provide and
what, if any, guarantees they can offer, before committing

**AVERAGE PRICE**
___

Variable, but as a
rule of thumb the
average cost of
products required
for a three-month
course of intensive
treatment would be
around
ῶ ῶ ῶ ῶ ῶ ῶ ῶ ῶ

yourself to such a highly priced regime.

## Minoxidil Treatment

Originally developed to reduce high blood pressure, Minoxidil is a drug-based treatment. In many countries, it can be obtained only through specialist hair-treatment centres, cosmetic-surgery clinics or, in some cases, on prescription from your doctor. Minoxidil is incorporated into lotion form which can be used at home. All the client has to do is apply the lotion topically to the scalp twice daily.

### Benefits and Claims
Providing the instructions are followed to the letter, a noticeable improvement can be expected after approximately four months.

### Results
Impossible to predict. Some clients have experienced a marked improvement in the growth and overall volume of their hair, while others have only attained minimal new growth or a fluffy down-like effect. The best results have been reported in younger men whose hair is thinning on the crown. Regardless of how little or how much growth you attain, if you want to maintain it, you will probably have to keep using Minoxidil for life, as the moment you stop you can expect to lose the lot.

### Value for Money?
Impossible to assess. As any results are unlikely to become apparent for at least four months, there is simply no way to predict whether this form of treatment will prove ultimately to be an expensive investment in disappointment, or a relatively cheap route to success.

**AVERAGE PRICE**

Per -Month
ῠ ῠ ῠ

### Warning Note
A number of products alleging to contain Minoxidil are

currently being offered for sale by mail order. In many countries it is illegal to advertise and sell drugs or medicines in this manner. If you are tempted to purchase any of these products, remember the rule of common law: *caveat emptor* – let the buyer beware, as, depending on how and where you purchase the product, you may not have any recourse to claiming a refund if the product fails to live up to its promise.

## Scalp Reduction

A quite drastic and painful procedure, scalp reduction involves removing a central section of the skin covering the crown and then pulling up, and suturing together, the two sections on either side of the head that still contain hair.

### Benefits and Claims
Reduces the size of the bald area or, if it is not too advanced, conceals it completely.

| AVERAGE PRICE |
| --- |
| Very expensive. |

### Results
Relatively permanent.

### Value for Money?
Impossible to evaluate on an objective basis.

## Trichological Treatments

Your first visit to a trichologist will involve an hour's consultation. During this time, the practitioner will take details of your medical history and of any genetic conditions that you or your parents might have in order to identify the likely cause of your hair problems. This will be followed by an examination of your scalp and hair with the aid of a trichogram.

In cases of MPB (see page 82), oestrogen-based creams applied topically to the scalp will help counteract the androgenic effect and prolong the hair's life and length. Other aids to treatment include steaming, vibro-massage and the use of ultraviolet and infra–red rays. A lotion will also be prescribed to be applied nightly at home. A treatment session will last approximately one hour, and these will initially need to be repeated weekly for a period of five or six weeks, reducing to fortnightly thereafter.

It is a strange but true fact that many countries still permit people to set themselves up as consultants or 'experts' in certain professional areas. These people are allowed to advertise their services, even if they have no relevant formal training or qualifications. Paradoxically, those who are most qualified are prevented, either by law or by their affiliation to a recognised professional institute or self-regulating association, from advertising either their existence or the professional services they offer. This crazy situation applies in the case of all trichologists (wherever in the world they practise) who are members of the Institute of Trichologists. To become a full member of the Institute involves spending three years studying such subjects as physics, chemistry, the function and use of electrical equipment, and the physiology and treatment of hair and scalp problems.

### Benefits and Claims
Helps slow down, and in some cases halt, MPB. It can successfully treat and resolve hair problems due to other causes.

### Results
Hair problems due to stress, childbirth, shock, nutritional deficiency and other causes usually respond successfully to treatment within approximately three months. For men suffering with MPB, the earlier preventive treatment is started, the more successful it is likely to be in slowing down hair loss. The average length of treatment for this condition is around five months, but in some cases maintenance treatments may be required for an indefinite period.

### Value for Money?
Excellent. Anyone suffering from any form of hair disorder

would be well-advised to consult a professional trichologist before exploring any other avenue of treatment. Seeking the advice of an acknowledged expert at the earliest opportunity can not only help safeguard against any further damage or hair loss, but could also potentially save you a lot of money and heartache in the long term.

A list of members of the Institute of Trichologists practising in your country or town can be obtained by sending a large, stamped addressed envelope to the Institute of Trichologists, 228 Stockwell Road, London SW9 9SU, England; telephone 071–733 2056.

| AVERAGE PRICE |
| :---: |
| Initial Consultation |
| Per treatment session – from |
| Take-home lotion |

## HOMOEOPATHY

On the face of it, homoeopathy may seem out of place in a book about beauty treatments. But if we accept the premise that true beauty can only be founded upon optimum health, then homoeopathy deserves its place here as an avenue worth exploring in the pursuit of outer beauty through the maintenance of inner harmony and health.

Homoeopathy was founded as a viable alternative to conventional medicine by a German physician, Samuel Hahnemann (1755–1843), who became increasingly concerned about the dangers and complications of many of the crude methods of treatment that were common in his day. The homoeopathic principle is best summed up by the Latin phrase, 'similia, similibus, curentus', meaning 'let like substances be used to treat like diseases'. A homoeopathic remedy is one that produces the same symptoms in a healthy person as those exhibited by the patient. Take, for example, belladonna, commonly known as deadly nightshade, the highly poisonous hedgerow plant. Belladonna is known to provoke a high, restless fever, thirst, irritability, and a burning, sore throat if ingested. When taken in its homoeopathic form, however, belladonna can be used as a curative for precisely these same symptoms.

An initial consultation with a homoeopath involves a very lengthy question-and-answer session. Apart from wanting to know every detail of the symptoms from which you are suffering, a homoeopath will also need to know everything about your medical history; appetite and diet; lifestyle; emotional and psychological states, and how these affect any symptoms; likes and dislikes; activities; hobbies; occupation; and the regularity of your bodily functions.

After assessing every one of these factors, and their bearing on your condition, the homoeopath will prescribe the correct remedy with which to begin treatment. Some homoeopaths dispense their own remedies, and charge accordingly; others will write out a prescription which can be taken to a homoeopathic pharmacist. He or she may also make a number of suggestions about alterations to your diet and lifestyle. A second consultation in order to interpret your response to treatment will follow a week or two later.

## Benefits and Claims

Homoeopathy is a safe, naturopathic form of medicine that is becoming increasingly popular as a method of treating the whole person, rather than the individual symptoms of an illness. It has been used successfully in treating a whole range of symptoms, conditions and diseases, from acne, asthma, eczema and eating disorders, to headaches, migraine, obesity and varicose veins. In fact, homoeopathic treatment can be fully effective in treating virtually any illness provided that there is no underlying mechanical or obstructive cause for its symptoms, such as a displacement of the spinal column or an obstruction of the bowel, which can only be relieved by manipulation or surgery.

The list of conditions that have been known to respond well to this form of treatment is so vast that it would be impossible to list them all here, yet it is important to stress that homoeopathy is not a cure-all. Rather it seeks to stimulate the immune system's own natural energies and defences to help heal itself and restore the body's own natural state of harmony and balance from within.

## Results

Some conditions of recent or non-chronic origin can be cleared up very quickly. Others may take considerably longer. In some cases it is quite common to find a different set of symptoms arising to replace those that have disappeared. Although this process of uncovering multi-layers of symptoms can be quite frustrating, it is nothing to be alarmed about. As long as you persevere with treatment according to your practitioner's advice, there is every chance that all your symptoms will eventually disappear.

## Value for Money?

Very good.

---

**AVERAGE PRICE**

Initial consultation
♨ ♨ ♨

Homoeopathic
remedies ♨

---

# HYDROTHERAPY

Water is the very essence of life. Not only is it fundamental to every living organism, but it also forms a high percentage of every vital organ and component in the human body. Water forms 90 per cent of our blood, 70 per cent of our skin, 80 per cent of our brain, and 25 per cent of our bones. The fact that water constitutes around 75 per cent of our body weight at birth, but only 50 per cent of it in later life is, according to many experts, a major cause of wrinkles in ageing skin.

In addition to being the best and most natural aid to physical health and beauty, water has inestimable benefits when applied externally to the body as a therapeutic treatment. The modern form of hydrotherapy developed gradually out of the pioneering work of Father Sebastian Kneipp. His famous and rigorous 'water cure' treatments included icy cold baths, showers, and walking barefoot in dewy grass, and were said to be responsible for restoring health and renewed vigour to many rich and titled clients who visited his famous 19th-century Bavarian spa.

Today's hydrotherapy treatments are based on scientifically established methods of applying water and a variety of

seaweeds, muds and herbs in order to achieve specific healing effects. The water and the herbal or mineral additives are
said to exert a stimulus on the body, which in turn creates a
physiological reaction within the body. This process improves
the circulation of blood to the surface tissues and the deep-
lying organs.

Water-therapy treatments have come a long way since
Kneipp's day. Underwater physiotherapy is proving to be an
invaluable aid in hospital treatments, and underwater therapies incorporating reflexology or deep-tissue massage are
becoming increasingly popular as a form of holistic health treatment in the United States. For many Europeans, however, by
far the greatest appeal of hydrotherapy lies in its alleged beau-
tifying/slimming effects.

There are almost as many variations on the theme of
hydrotherapy as a beauty treatment as there are manufacturers specialising in this area. Predominantly, however, the
majority of these treatments can be separated into two distinct
types: those that involve immersion in a tub containing certain
recommended ingredients, and those that require the client
to stand while being hosed down by a water cannon. In order
to avoid boring the reader with a list of lengthy and largely
repetitive descriptions of what are essentially similar treatments marketed under different brand names, I have confined
this section to providing an overview of the differences that
exist between these two main types.

## Hydrotherapy Baths

Most hydrotherapy baths will involve an all-over body scrub,
followed by immersion in a tub of warm or hot water containing mineral-rich substances such as micronised marine algae,
Dead-Sea mineral salts, seaweed extracts, volcanic muds,
aromatherapy oils, or a mixture of ingredients derived from
herbs and plants. These are said to remineralise the body,
restore lost trace elements to the skin, accelerate circulation,
improve muscle tone, and generally assist in the weight-loss

process by aiding the breakdown of fatty deposits and speeding up the elimination of toxins.

After being immersed in the special tub for 10 minutes or so, a number of water inlets placed at strategic points will be activated to allow tiny jets of water through to pummel and massage the body. The therapist will then use a special hose attachment to massage specific muscle groups by directing a strong jet of water slowly back and forth across your upright body for between 5 and 10 minutes. This will be followed by a further 10 minutes or so relaxing in the tub with the tiny jets switched on to provide a gentler pummelling. Once this is complete, you will be assisted out of the bath, towelled off, and given a whole body massage.

### Benefits and Claims
Hot-water or steam therapy helps dilate the blood vessels, lowers blood pressure, relaxes muscles and joints, induces sweating, sedates the system and enhances sleep.

### Results
You will feel rejuvenated, invigorated, refreshed, toned, sleek and squeaky-clean. One session is not sufficient to contribute to any inch-loss or weight-loss but, taken regularly, a hydrotherapy bath treatment can be a useful adjunct to a new get-slim-and-healthy regime.

### Value for Money?
Despite the fact that this is both marginally less invigorating and slightly more expensive than the hydrotherapy 'hosing' treatment (see page 96), the overall effect on body contour and skin condition is more or less the same. The added benefit of the whole-body massage makes this pretty good value for money.

| AVERAGE PRICE |
| :---: |
| ♆ ♆ ♆ |

## Hydrotherapy 'Hosing' Treatments

This type of treatment requires the client to stand naked (apart from a shower cap and a pair of protective goggles) at one end of a narrow tiled tunnel facing a therapist who is armed with a hose. Then a strong jet of water that hits you with the force of a cannon is played slowly back and forth over the body in a controlled sequence of movements. This cold-water technique is specifically aimed at stimulating the lymphatic system and encouraging the breakdown of fatty deposits. Once the initial shock has worn off, you soon become acclimatised to the variations that take place in the pressure and temperature of the water. The overall sensation is rather like being subjected to an incredible massage with an alternating rhythm of firm pummelling and gentle kneading.

### Benefits and Claims
Helps smoothen fatty lumps of tissue to reshape the figure. Tests show that cold-water therapy can reduce inflammation and congestion on the surface of the skin, increase the circulation of blood and oxygen to the internal organs, stimulate respiration, tone the muscles, and increase the metabolic rate by as much as 80 per cent.

### Results
Depending on the state and condition of your body, you may not notice any discernible difference after just one treatment, although you will feel incredibly clean and invigorated. While the recommended course is six or twelve treatments, most people usually begin to notice some toning and firming effect after the second or third. At the end of a course, your clothes will be a little looser, and your body will feel tighter and more conditioned. Results will be far less noticeable on the obese, or those who are already fairly slim and/or firmly-toned.

It is fairly common to experience a degree of light-headedness at the start of treatment, while those with cellulite may notice some tenderness and bruising in these areas.

### Value for Money?
Taken as a pre-holiday or post-diet toning treatment – yes. It

could also be worth it purely for the sheer feeling of vitality and glowing good health it imparts.

## INCH-LOSS TREATMENTS

We all *know* that it is impossible to dissolve fat instantly, and that miracle cures to weight problems simply do not exist. Despite this, however, the majority of us still cling on to the hope that somehow, some day, some enterprising scientist or chemist will answer our prayers by inventing the ultimate, guaranteed 100 per cent effective panacea for superfluous fat.

While most of us can accept, at least on an intellectual level, that slenderness does not necessarily equate with success or happiness, the myriad inferences to the contrary that assault us daily are a powerful influence on our emotions and our psyche. Consequently, few of us are immune to the sugges- tion that if we were only to try this amazing new machine or that truly wonderful new treatment, our prayers would be answered. The sad truth is, though, that they rarely are. But the prospect of rapid reduction nonetheless retains its power to lure us on, regardless of all the disappointments we may have encountered in the past. And the more susceptible we become, the more the slimming industry expands.

Today, virtually every high street in every town boasts a salon or health club touting its own particular version of the ultimate inch-loss body wrap or treatment. There are so many of these that reviewing each and every variation would alone take far more months of research than my team and I had at our disposal. Moreover, as so many of these treatments are very similar, I have not listed every single brand or version. I have instead limited this section to providing an overview of a few of the more popular brands of treatments currently avail- able, on the basis that, while certain aspects of the specific processes used may vary, the underlying principles and effects are largely the same. Similarly, rather than risk repeating certain comments pertaining to the likely value-for-money factor involved with each treatment, it seemed more sensible to offer a collective, but *generalised*, assessment at the end of this section.

The majority of inch-loss treatments fall into one of two categories – those that incorporate the use of electrical gadgets or faradic-current machines as an integral part of the treatment, and those that rely solely on a combination of 'natural' ingredients and tight body wrapping to produce the desired effect.

## Body Wraps

The use of body wraps is not a new idea. Cleopatra is alleged to have used them regularly to maintain the condition of her figure and skin, while the therapeutic benefits of applying hot poultices and cold compresses to affected parts of the body have been recorded in medical treatises dating back thousands of years.

### Finders Inch Wrap

> **AVERAGE PRICE**
>
> Full-body treatment
> Ⓤ Ⓤ Ⓤ Ⓤ
>
> Hip and thighs only
> – from Ⓤ Ⓤ

This two-hour treatment commences with a detailed discussion and notation of your medical history and current problems. Next, your entire body is exfoliated from neck to feet and a careful note is made of all your measurements. This is followed by a massage with a Dead-Sea mineral-rich moisturising cream and the application of several layers of plastic food wrapping which is wound tightly around the body to seal in the cream. Garmented like a mummy in acres of clingfilm, with a terry towelling jumpsuit worn on top for good measure, you will be left alone to relax for the duration of the treatment.

### Benefits and Claims

Removes dry, dead skin cells, improves suppleness and texture of the skin, detoxifies the system and helps with inch loss on strategic areas which are prone to fat build-up.

### Inchwrap

Two hours of treatment remarkably similar to that described

above. The only difference here is that the 'active solution' looks like some form of mud.

## Benefits and Claims

All the above-mentioned benefits, plus a claim that the effects should last for a month... with the aid of three home products! One treatment per month is recommended.

## Slimwrap

The therapist begins by taking detailed measurements of your ankles, calves, knees, thighs, bottom, hips and waist, and marking the position of the tape measure. He or she then commences to wrap your torso and each limb carefully in bandages soaked in a special solution claimed to be rich in vitamins and minerals. When the wrapping process is complete – this can easily take 10–15 minutes – a plastic sauna suit has to be worn over the top to help the body absorb the solution. No further effort is required; you simply lie down and relax as the suit, the solution, and the bandage compress encourage the excess inches to melt magically away.

At the end of the session, the tape measure is placed at the pre-marked positions, and every fraction of an inch lost is recorded on a card. When totalled up and given as a combined figure, the amount of inches lost overall can sound very impressive.

## Benefits and Claims

One treatment is said to result in a considerable loss of inches (anything from 10–20 or more has been quoted). Any loss is claimed to be permanent – provided that you are careful about what you eat and drink. For best results, a course of six treatments is recommended.

## Universal Contour Wrap

This treatment, which lasts for two-and-a-half hours, involves being covered in a solution of sea clay. Elastic bandages and a vinyl sauna suit complete the ensemble. Instead of being left

---

**AVERAGE PRICE**

Whole-body
treatment 💋 💋 💋 💋

Set of three home
products – from
💋 💋

---

**AVERAGE PRICE**

Single treatment
💋 💋 💋
Course of 6 – from
💋 💋 💋 💋 💋 💋

to relax, the remaining treatment time is spent exercising on a series of toning tables.

### Benefits and Claims
Increases circulation, helps to disperse cellulite, and improves the condition of the skin. A noticeable reduction in measurements.

### Results
The fundamental misconception we commonly make is to equate inch loss with fat loss. While there is no denying that a body-wrap treatment will result in an immediate and measurable reduction in bodily dimensions, it is very important not to confuse this with a reduction in body *fat*. A single body-wrap treatment will have a short-term effect on the amount of fluid that is retained in the body. The results may last for 24 hours, or for anything up to seven days, but there are no guarantees as so much depends on each person's lifestyle.

That is not to say, however, that body-wrap treatments are a total waste of time and money, for they do have their uses. Firstly, the temporary inch loss can be a real incentive at the start of a new diet. Secondly, they are better than a shoe horn for helping you to wriggle into a tight-fitting dress on special occasions when you really want to look your best. And thirdly, a course of treatments can be very beneficial in helping to kick-start a sluggish circulation, detoxify the system and aid the lymphatic drainage process, all of which are vital for optimum health and vitality. But *only* if you are determined to make the necessary changes to your diet and lifestyle.

**AVERAGE PRICE**

Single treatment
♉ ♉ ♉ ♉
(slight reduction on booking the recommended course of three).

### Value for Money?
If you want a short-term answer to a long-term problem, a single treatment of any of the above represents reasonable value for money. If you are looking for a permanent solution, and are prepared to invest extra effort to back up the treatment by exercising regularly, sticking to a diet that is low in salt, sugar and fat, cutting out smoking and alcohol, and drink-

ing plenty of water, then a course could potentially prove to be excellent value for money. Otherwise, do not bother.

## Electrical Treatments

Most electrical inch-loss treatments are based on the principle of faradism (electrical muscle stimulation). By causing the muscles to contract and relax unaided by the client, these machines are claimed to provide the same tightening and toning effects you would get from isometric exercise without the effort involved. In some cases a body-wrap process is also incorporated to boost circulation and enhance the eliminatory effects.

As the majority of treatments that fall into this category appear to offer a more positive and, in many cases, longer-lasting solution for those wishing to reduce their size, this section provides an individual evaluation of the results and potential value-for-money factor of each treatment.

### Arasys

Born out of the 'new-wave' in advanced beauty treatments, Arasys could almost be described as a 'son of Slendertone', insofar as it shares many of its worthy predecessor's principles and features. It is claimed, however, to be distinguishable by benefit of a few technological refinements of its own. Instead of spending 30 minutes or an hour of your valuable time being strapped, padded and connected via a series of electrodes to one of the old-style muscle-toning machines, the 'more efficient and effective smooth-topped faradic wave form' unique to Arasys is said to ensure bigger and better effects in a mere quarter of that time.

If you have ever tried a Slendertone treatment, then you will know broadly what to expect. Your measurements will be recorded before and after the first, fifth and final treatments. Rubber pads are strapped to the areas requiring toning, firming, or reducing, the machine is set, and for the next 15 minutes a series of strong, rhythmic electrical pulses will stimulate the muscles continuously to contract and relax. There is no need for the therapist to remain with you as a hand-held cancellation switch is – reassuringly – supplied. I say 'reassuringly' because one can only give a subjective interpretation of the degree of discomfort involved; the reports I have received vary from 'a mild tingling' sensation' and 'slightly uncomfortable' all the way up to 'so unbearable I wouldn't want to repeat it'. And as the current gets stronger with each successive treatment, this could prove to be an important factor.

## Benefits and Claims

- Firms and tones the muscles.
- Increases the metabolic rate.
- Improves circulation to help remove toxins and break down cellulite and body fat.
- Reduces inches.
- Creates a feeling of extra energy and well-being.
- One 15-minute session on the bottom is said to equal 400 strenuous buttock raises, while a course of 10 is said to have a lasting result.

## Results

These can be quite impressive. One tester reported a noticeable difference in firming up, but no visible difference in cellulite, after just four treatments. Another claimed to have lost a total of 10 inches overall after a course of 10 sessions. A third said her course had resulted in a higher and tighter bottom plus a slimmer waist and thighs.

## Value for Money?

If you need toning up but cannot stand the thought of exercise, or do not have time to visit a gym regularly, then this could be money well spent. While the overall price is reasonable enough, however, three sessions a week could make a sizeable hole in the average woman's purse — but if you do not mind paying this price for your inertia the results that are potentially achievable could make this a worthwhile investment.

On the down side, the treatment will not necessarily make you any fitter, and it can only resculpt and tone one area of your body at a time. Thus, not only may you need more than 10 treatments to achieve the overall result you are looking for but, if you have no intention of changing your lifestyle, you also may need to commit yourself to a regular programme of maintenance treatments. Either way, the cost could be considerably higher than your initial estimate.

Overall, however, if you are looking for maximum results with minimum effort, Arasys is one form of treatment that is definitely worth considering.

**AVERAGE PRICE**

Single session –
from **♉**

Recommended
course of 10
**♉ ♉ ♉ ♉ ♉ ♉**

### Fisiotron

Described as an 'individual body contouring system', Fisiotron incorporates a combination of aromatherapy oils and creams with electrical stimulation of the muscles to achieve an improvement in cellulite and a reduction in body size. Some salons offer a special package that also includes an additional session with massage and G5 treatment to enhance the effects of Fisiotron.

Offered on its own, a Fisiotron treatment consists of a number of stages and takes 45 minutes overall. At your initial treatment, the first stage will involve taking measurements at precise intervals between your ankle and chest. This stage will be repeated again at the commencement of your fifth and tenth (last) treatment so that a running check can be kept on the total number of inches lost overall. The actual measuring device, which is said to be unique to Fisiotron, consists of a master tape secured to a base plate which is run up the left side and down the right side of the body. Sixteen separate tapes are then attached at intervals to record the girth of specific areas.

The next stage involves an exfoliating scrub and the application of a combination of specially formulated aromatherapy oils and creams. These are said to help eliminate fluid retention and toxins, stimulate lymph and blood circulation, tone up the skin and underlying tissue, and break down fatty deposits. Next, the body is wrapped from neck to ankle in elasticated bandages, which will have been pre-soaked in hot water, to aid conduction. A number of black graphite straps leading from the Fisiotron computer are then connected to your body through which electrical currents flow to your muscles causing them to contract and relax. The computer is claimed to be able to react and adjust the treatment in accordance with each client's individual condition. Once the machine has been disconnected and the bandages removed, more creams are applied to further improve the circulation and condition of the skin.

## Benefits and Claims

The manufacturers are emphatic that Fisiotron does not reduce poundage, but they say it can and does achieve a reduction of body size – up to two dress sizes – during a short course of treatment. They also claim that, unlike other treatments that remove water from the body temporarily, Fisiotron can actually clear the drainage system (almost like de-furring a kettle, they say) so that the body can continue to remove excess fluid and waste products in the way that nature intended.

## Results

Definite improvements in skin and body tone and a reduction in inches have been recorded by several testers – some of whom noticed a marked difference after only two treatments. Whether the results last is debatable, as a lot depends on individual lifestyle factors. Some salons recommend an annual follow-up course, while others say that a mini-course twice-yearly is sufficient to maintain results.

## Value for Money?

If you can afford it, this is definitely worth trying.

**AVERAGE PRICE**

Single treatment –
from 𝓤 𝓤

Course of 10 – from
𝓤 𝓤 𝓤 𝓤 𝓤 𝓤 𝓤
(if massage and G5
treatment are
included you can
expect to pay a
little more).

## Frigi Thalgo Seaweed Body Treatment

Seaweed and marine algae have long been thought to contain powerful slimming and diuretic properties. Thalgo were one of the first companies to incorporate marine extracts into their beauty-treatment range.

This one-hour treatment, which is designed to 'intensively refine and firm the silhouette', commences with the usual measuring process, plus an all-over body scrub to remove dead skin cells. As with most other body treatments, the position of the tape measure is marked against the skin so that the resulting inch loss can be assessed accurately. Each leg is wrapped individually in cold bandages soaked in a seaweed and camphor solution to help promote localised fluid loss, and then wired up to a faradic exercise machine for 20 minutes or so. This is followed by an invigorating massage to further stimulate the circulation and aid the removal of excess fluid and toxins.

### Benefits and Claims

- Detoxifies the body.
- Stimulates circulation.
- Improves overall skin tone.
- Helps eliminate toxins.
- Promotes localised fluid and inch loss.

### Results

Smoother skin, better muscle tone, and the disappearance of a few unwanted inches.

### Value for Money?

As this is not noticeably any more effective than other similar treatments, it is hard to justify its higher price.

| AVERAGE PRICE |
| :---: |
| Single treatment |
| 🌷🌷🌷 |
| Course of 6 – from |
| 🌷🌷🌷🌷🌷🌷 |

## Ionithermie

One of the older, more established names in inch-loss treatments, Ionithermie combines the benefits of a body wrap with passive faradic exercise. A one-hour treatment kicks off with the usual measuring process, and a massage with special creams and toners. Layers of damp muslin soaked in clay are applied to the body from the waist down, and electrical pads are then attached, through which galvanic and faradic currents pass. The faradic current stimulates the contraction and relaxation of muscles, while the galvanic current is used to propel the active ingredients contained in the cream deep into the skin.

## Benefits and Claims

Immediate inch loss (which is claimed to last 'indefinitely'), improved skin tone and texture, and a noticeable improvement in cellulite. Best results are claimed to be achieved with a course of five sessions taken at fortnightly intervals, topped up by the use of home products, and a follow-up treatment every second month thereafter.

## Results

There is a great deal of variation in the results obtained by different testers. Some said there was a discernible difference in their cellulite; others claimed not to notice any difference at all; but all did indeed experience an immediate, albeit temporary, inch loss.

## Value for Money?

Although this falls into the category of being a useful, emergency aid for helping you squeeze into a tight-fitting dress when the need arises, you would have to be pretty desperate, or pretty cavalier with your money to favour this over one of its cheaper competitors. Moreover, at this price level, one ought to be able to anticipate better long-term effects. As all the evidence seems to point to the contrary, it fails to meet my criterion for a 'good value-for-money' treatment.

AVERAGE PRICE
_____

Single treatment –
from
🌷🌷

Recommended
course of 5 –
treatments
🌷🌷🌷🌷🌷🌷

## Transion

Yet another variation on the theme of muscle-toning inch-loss treatments based solely on passive exercise.

## Benefits and Claims

All the usual, but with a refreshing touch of honesty thrown in – you are actually told that the results are only likely to last for up to 10 days, although the more treatments you have, the more toned-up your muscles will become.

## Results

Temporary inch loss, but both the results and the duration of its effects are said to accumulate with a recommended course of 10 treatments taken twice weekly.

## Value for Money?

Minimal.

| AVERAGE PRICE |
| :---: |
| Single 30-minute treatment 🌷 |
| Recommended course of 10 – from 🌷🌷🌷🌷 |

## Ultraslim

Works on precisely the same principles as all the other treatments that rely solely on faradism for their results.

## Benefits and Claims

All the usual – and did you know that 17 minutes of average intensity treatment to your stomach muscles is equivalent to 12,000-15,000 sit-ups? Or so they claim. As usual, a course of 10 treatments is recommended.

## Results

Depends upon one's perception but, according to several testers' reports, there can be a big difference between your own assessment of any inch loss, and that recorded by some therapists.

## Value for Money?

Minimal.

# LAUGHTER THERAPY

| AVERAGE PRICE |
| :---: |
| Single treatment – |
| **ᵾ ᵾ** |

What does laughter therapy have to do with beauty treatments? A lot more than you might think! Although this is one treatment that is not included on any beauty salon's list, it is worthy of its place in this book for two reasons. Firstly, laughter is now being hailed as one of the most effective health-and-beauty treatments that has ever been invented; and secondly, when it comes to value for money, it outstrips virtually every other treatment on the market, not only because there are enormous life-enhancing (and even life-prolonging) benefits attached to laughter, but also because it is very often free.

Despite the fact that this may sound like a contradiction in terms, laughter is now being taken very seriously indeed. The results of more than 100 scientific studies have shown that, not only is laughter extremely good for your looks (laughing exercises far more facial muscles than frowning), but it is also remarkably beneficial for the body.

According to American cardiologist, Dr William Fry, one minute of laughter has an effect on the body equivalent to 40 minutes of relaxation. In fact, so seriously is this information being taken that some American hospitals now have 'humour rooms' where patients are encouraged to read funny comics and watch side-splitting videos to help speed their recovery from operations and illness.

Even the British medical professional now deems laughter therapy to be worthy of further investigation and experimentation. In 1992, the first National Health Service-funded laughter clinic was established in the midlands city of Birmingham by laughter therapist and stress consultant, Robert Holden. In addition to publishing a book on the subject, Holden also runs a series of workshops and courses in laughter medicine for professionals. Says Holden, who first discovered the healing power of laughter when working with people who suffered from stress-related illness, 'People can spend hours talking about a problem, but ask them to talk about something joyful for five minutes and they are stuck for words.'

## Benefits and Claims

Laughter relaxes the body by reducing muscle tension and blood pressure. It also stimulates the production and release of endorphins into the bloodstream, which relieve stress and pain. Science now recognises that endorphins are responsible for creating the natural 'high' we experience whenever we are feeling extra happy. Moreover, endorphins can also reduce illness, control stress and promote good health.

Misery is a vicious cycle. Unhappiness creates tension, which has a negative effect on posture and digestion and which, in turn, causes pain and discomfort. The resulting effects are felt in the body as stress which, as we all know by now, can pose such a serious threat to our health that it is often cited as a major contributory factor to many killer diseases.

Even in its mildest form, stress can radiate its effects through-out the entire system. Apart from putting pressure on the internal organs, it reflects itself externally on the face. And all it takes to spark off this negative feedback loop is one single, solitary, unhappy thought. Conversely, science has proven that the mere action of lifting up the corners of the mouth in a smile – even if the smile is false – can create a positive-feed-back loop that has tremendous benefits – psychologically, emotionally and physically. Being unable to distinguish a genuine smile from a false one, the brain reacts to both by releasing precisely the same chemicals into the bloodstream.

## Results

Smiles and laughter make us feel and look better. Happiness and laughter are contagious; they draw other people towards us like a magnet, and they make even the plainest person look and feel beautiful. Moreover, people who laugh readily, and who have an optimistic outlook on life, not only live longer and healthier lives, they also come out top in surveys seeking to establish the most desirable and attractive qualities in the opposite sex.

**AVERAGE PRICE**

Robert Holden's Laughter Workshop – from 🌷🌷

Robert Holden's book, *Laughter: The Best Medicine?* (Thorsons) 🌷

Laughter therapy is also available free from a variety of other sources.

### Value for Money?

Undeniably one of the best value-for-money health and beauty treatments in this book. For details of Robert Holden's Laughter Clinic and Workshops telephone: 021–551 2932.

## LYMPHATIC DRAINAGE

Lymph is a watery mixture made up partly of liquid plasma of the blood, and partly of fluid produced by the body cells it bathes. It travels through a series of vessels known as the lymphatic system, and has a two-fold function – it carries dissolved nutrients from the blood through the walls of the capillaries to the body's tissues, and acts as a drainage system to collect and carry dissolved waste products from the tissues back to the blood on its return journey.

Factors that can contribute to poor lymphatic drainage include lack of exercise, poor circulation, inadequate nutrition and an overload of toxins in the body from alcohol, drugs, tobacco and environmental pollution. Once the free flow of the body's waste-disposal system becomes impeded, stagnation occurs. Toxins and water build up and the membranes around the fat cells harden and become lumpy. This in turn leads to a build-up of fatty tissue and, ultimately, cellulite.

There are a number of methods for stimulating a sluggish lymphatic system. Exercise helps, as this increases the circulation and the rate of blood and lymph flow. Massage can also be useful in encouraging the movement of stored toxins towards the body's natural purification centres. Fasts and elimination diets can be used in conjunction with dry-skin brushing to encourage the elimination of toxic matter trapped in the body's tissues, and certain aromatherapy oils known for their detoxifying effects can help improve the situation.

Although most of the treatments covered in the section on cellulite claim also to *aid* lymphatic drainage, there appears to be only one form of mechanical treatment on the market at the moment that concentrates specifically on this problem.

As this form of treatment, which is based upon a device that was originally used in hospitals, is currently being marketed and promoted under two separate product names, the comments outlined below should be taken to apply in both cases.

## Aromazone and Normaform Lymphatic Drainage Systems

This half-hour treatment involves sitting or lying on a salon couch with your feet and legs inserted into a long pair of inflatable, pressurised 'boots' attached to an electrically operated machine. When the machine is switched on, the boots inflate. The build-up of pressure flows over the limbs in a gentle, gripping and relaxing wave-like motion designed to mimic the pumping action of the muscles, creating an odd, but not necessarily unpleasant sensation.

By far the oddest thing about this form of treatment, however, is that when the inflatable 'boots' are removed, they reveal the imprint of a clearly defined network of raised lines on your legs which can remain for anything up to an hour afterwards. These lines, which tend to look just like the imprint of 'veins' discernible on a leaf, are said to be the raised lymph vessels; the more visible they are, the more effective the treatment is claimed to have been. Although it is only the legs that are massaged, the treatment is said to work on the entire lymphatic drainage system to benefit the whole of the body.

### Benefits and Claims

- Increases circulation.
- Stimulates efficient lymphatic drainage.
- Helps detoxify the body.
- Improves the appearance of the skin on the face and body.
- Aids in the elimination of cellulite.

### Results

Inconclusive as a single treatment, but can accelerate and enhance the process of lymphatic drainage when regular treatments are combined with other measures such as exercise and a detoxification diet.

AVERAGE PRICE

ꊶ ꊶ

## Value for Money?
Pricey, but could be worthwhile for its overall long-term benefits.

# MAGNET THERAPY

This natural therapy is based on the theory that electromagnetic forces can be used to correct imbalances within the body. Although most of the supportive evidence is largely empirical, and therefore unsubstantiated according to scientific codes of practice, this should not necessarily be taken to mean that this theory is totally without foundation.

Magnet therapy has been around for a very long time. According to historical documents, it was a popular method of pain-relieving treatment among the ancient Greeks, and Cleopatra is said to have worn a magnet on her forehead in order to preserve her beauty.

As increasing numbers of people are rejecting conventional drug therapy for alternative methods of treatment, more and more alternative practitioners are incorporating the use of magnet therapy. It is used not only to relieve pain, but also to provide a more natural form of treatment to help alleviate a wide range of ailments from headaches and migraines to conditions such as ulcers, arthritis and asthma. For some years now, magnetic plasters have been widely available in health shops and pharmacies throughout continental Europe and America. These can be used by the purchaser to alleviate pain caused by arthritis, rheumatism, migraine and menstruation.

Holistic therapist Bharti Vyas is the first British practitioner to offer magnet therapy as both a health and beauty treatment at her Holistic Therapy Beauty Centre, and also the first to incorporate magnets into a DIY home face-lifting kit. According to Vyas, 'Magnets are as natural as nature itself.

The Earth is a huge magnet and possesses its own magnetic field, as we all do within it. Since our bodies are surrounded by a sea of magnetic waves, it is therefore not only possible, but entirely natural, that magnets could have a positive and restorative influence on our health.'

Treatment is based on placing the magnets on acupressure points of the face, with special emphasis on the jowl area. After massaging a therapy oil into the skin, one magnet is placed on either side of the nose, and just below the corners of the mouth. Plasters are applied to hold the magnets in position, and they should then be left in place for a minimum of six hours while you sleep.

### Benefits and Claims
Magnet therapy revolves around the two magnetic poles. Placing the north pole against the body is said to have a stimulating and energising effect, while the south pole is claimed to have a calming and suppressive influence.

### Results
After just one treatment, you can distinctly feel and see a slight lifting in the area of the jowls. One tester who tried the magnets out for a period of several weeks claimed they not only made her face and skin feel better, but they made a definite improvement to the appearance of her face.

During a visit to a major health exhibition in the United States, I tried magnet therapy for myself. Footsore and weary, I was invited by one exhibitor to sit myself down, remove my shoes and spend five minutes relaxing with a magnetic necklace wrapped around my feet. Within moments I was aware of a strange tingling sensation. Five minutes later my feet felt as refreshed and revitalised as they had at the beginning of the day. I was so impressed, I bought one!

On returning home, I subjected magnet therapy to another small test. I wrapped the necklace around my sister-in-law's wrist to see what effect it might have on alleviating a long-standing rheumatic condition that habitually caused much

**AVERAGE PRICE**

Bharti Vyas'
Magnetic Face-
Lifting Kit

🌷🌷🌷🌷

stiffness and aching in her hand. Within 15 minutes she, too, reported feeling the same tingling sensation I had experienced. An hour later she was able to flex her fingers quite freely, and all the aching had gone. Despite returning the necklace to me before she went home, her hand, wrist and fingers remained flexible and pain-free for a further 24 hours.

### Value for Money?

Taking into account all the health and beauty benefits associated with magnet therapy, and therefore the potential other uses to which this kit can be put, overall it represents very good value for money.

### Warning

Magnet therapy should not be used by heart patients and people fitted with pacemakers.

## MANICURES AND NAIL TREATMENTS

Hands and nails are one of the most used and abused parts of the human body. Just like our faces, they are constantly exposed to the elements. Sun, wind, water and detergents are unavoidable realities of modern life. While our skin is a marvellous organ that provides all-over protection, the fact that we have only a relatively thin covering of it over our hands and fingers means that these areas are far more vulnerable to premature wrinkling. There are three main reasons why hands are probably the biggest 'giveaway' to our true age. Firstly, because they contain far less fat than our faces, they are particularly prone to ageing. Secondly, the underlying muscle mass, which is not too plentiful to begin with, begins to diminish and atrophy with age, which only exacerbates the claw-like effect created by protruding tendons and veins. And thirdly, because oil production is skimpier in the back of our hands, the skin here is far more prone to dehydration and flaking.

Apart from moisturising the hands daily and wearing rubber

gloves to protect them whenever they need to be immersed
in water, regular manicures can provide essential protection
to your hands and nails. After years of stagnation as a stand-
by salon treatment, today's new crop of manicures are proving
responsible for opening up a whole new area in niche
marketing; one which is affording numerous self-employment
opportunities for women seeking to operate their own
business.

Every manicurist has her own favourite techniques for hand
and nail care. Some incorporate hand reflexology techniques
in their treatments; others rely on the use of aromatherapy.
But by far the most exciting aspect of the manicure business
is the sheer range and choice of innovative nail treatments that
are constantly being developed as a result of the latest scientific research.

According to one recent magazine report, some manufacturers are experimenting with nail polishes containing Kevlar
– a substance used in the fibres of bulletproof vests and fire-
fighter's boots – in the hope of creating the ultimate varnish,
guaranteed to make even weak nails rock-hard. Moreover,
specialists in a New York hospital are said to be conducting
exhaustive tests on a number of new hair-stimulating drugs as
part of a research programme specifically aimed at discovering how to stimulate and accelerate nail growth.

Meanwhile, thanks to the new science of nail cosmetology,
which is continually devising new and vastly superior formulas to create stronger, longer, and more realistic nail tips and
extensions, the false-nail business is enjoying an unprecedented
boom.

## Nail Tips

These can be affixed to your own nails to give an impression
of length. For best results, your own nail should extend at
least a few millimetres beyond your fingertip. A special adhe-
sive is used to glue the tips to your natural nail, and the surface
is filed down to conceal the join.

## Built-up Tips

A specially formed piece of plastic or a thin, flexible piece of metal is inserted beneath your existing nail. This extends beyond the tip of your own nail to provide a mould. Then a special acrylic mixture is painted on top of your own nail and upwards over the form. Once the mixture has hardened and dried, the form is removed, leaving behind a built-up tip which can be filed to the desired shape and length. As the acrylic mixture is transparent, the nails can either be left 'nude' or painted with a coloured varnish.

## Nail Wraps

Nail wraps are used as a strengthening treatment for weak nails. This involves applying a thin layer of finely woven silk 'webbing' to the nail and gluing it into place. After filing away any excess material from the edges, the nails are usually painted with a few coats of polish in order both to cover up the slightly rough surface appearance of the nail and also to create additional protection.

## Light Concept Nails

Light bonding is one of the latest innovations in nail technology. Using a range of new synthetic materials (reactive acrylesters) the Light Concept Nail system consists of a combined bonder, sculptor and sealant in a gel formula. This is suitable for creating extensions, and for adding to existing nails either as a strengthener or to fill in depressions. The gel also contains a special curing glass fibre which hardens very quickly when exposed to ultraviolet light.

### Benefits and Claims

Regular manicure treatments are claimed to help improve the condition of the skin on your hands, and strengthen and shape the nails. Fake-nail systems claim to create realistic-looking, long, sculptured fingernails that will not crack, chip or flake. Most fake-nail systems also claim to last for several weeks.

## Results
In the hands of a good therapist, regular manicures usually achieve a significant improvement in the appearance and condition of your hands and nails. All the above fake-nail systems look good when first applied. The only difference is that some are tougher, more resilient and longer-lasting than others. Precisely how long they last depends on your lifestyle and the degree of wear and tear to which you subject your hands.

## Value for Money?
Overall, pretty good.

---

**AVERAGE PRICE**

Normal manicure treatment 🌷🌷

Special manicure treatments, e.g. those involving reflexology or aromatherapy massage 🌷🌷

Fake tips, extension and light-bonding nail treatments – between 🌷🌷 and 🌷🌷🌷

---

# MARY COHR CATIOVITAL FACIAL TREATMENT

Mary Cohr is a sister company launched and presided over personally by J.D. Mondin, the current head of René Guinot. A doctor in pharmaceutics, Mondin is alleged to have developed his own research programme in collaboration with major hospitals and universities. Any discoveries resulting from this research is then incorporated into the range of treatments, products and innovations marketed under the Mary Cohr name.

Catiovital is a four-phase facial treatment designed and formulated by Mondin specifically for mature skin. Phase one of this two-hour treatment session commences with a thorough cleansing of the skin, prior to the application of a preheated, see-through gauze mask. The warmth of the mask, and the active principles used in conjunction with it, are designed to create a sauna-like effect to help open the pores and free them of ingrained make-up, sebum and atmospheric pollutants.

In phase two, the therapist treats any specific skin problems such as dryness, fine lines and spots by applying the appropriate ionisable gel and gently massaging it into the skin with the aid of two flat-ended metal rods through which a galvanic current passes.

Phase three consists of nourishing the skin through massage with essential oils selected specially to suit your own skin type. And phase four involves the application of a relaxing mask followed by a protective day or night cream.

### Benefits and Claims

Helps replenish vital ingredients necessary for a healthy complexion, and protect the skin against further damage. Immediate visible difference in the condition, tone and brightness of the complexion, which improves progressively with regular treatment. For best results, one treatment every four to six weeks is recommended.

### Results

Having tried this particular treatment myself, I can only agree with other testers who rate it as one of the most relaxing and impressive facial treatments currently available. After spending months testing a variety of the latest anti-ageing products and treatments on my own face, I did not need the therapist to tell me that my skin, which is not normally dry, was suffering from a bad case of dehydration. After just one treatment, there was a marked improvement in the tone, texture and condition of my skin – it literally glowed with health.

### Value for Money?

As a remedial or preventive treatment, this is well worth every penny.

## MARY COHR EYE TECH

Invented by Artistic Director, Michel Limongi, in response to repeated requests from women desperate to change the shape of their eyes, Eye Tech is an ingenious alternative to cosmetic surgery for those whose droopy, crepey eyelids make them look tired, sad or prematurely old. Designed to be placed in the crease of the upper eye, Eye Tech consists of a set of virtually invisible, hypo-allergenic, flesh-coloured micro-strips which create a lifting action on the eye contour itself. Because the strips are so fine, and made from a 'breathable' material, they should remain in place for anything up to a week. They are said to mould like a second skin, and be virtually undetectable, even at close quarters.

Although Eye Tech can be purchased over the counter at some salons and department stores, it is advisable to have your therapist apply them in the first instance, so that she can demonstrate precisely how they should be worn for the best effect. They come in a special mirrored case containing 18 pairs, and they can be worn with or without make-up.

## Benefits and Claims

- Transforms the appearance of the eyes.
- Creates a more youthful, wide-eyed look.

## Results

Although they are a bit tricky to get the hang of, once applied properly they really do make a difference to the appearance and shape of your eyes. A brilliant alternative to surgery.

## Value for Money?

Provided that you do not waste too many strips in your attempts to fit them in precisely the right place, they provide very good value for money. Do make sure, however, that your therapist knows how to apply them properly and explains the technique clearly to you. One tester who made a special trip to a leading department store to try them out was initially very disappointed, but once she had been shown how to use them correctly, she thought they were the best thing to be invented since sliced bread! Coming from someone who was seriously

**AVERAGE PRICE**

Initial consultation and box of 18 Eye Tech strips 🌷 🌷

Refills 🌷

considering having surgery on her eyelids, this is praise indeed.

# MARY COHR LIFTING-BEAUTÉ

Described as the nearest salon equivalent to a face-lift, this treatment is based on a combination of collagen, DNA and liposomes. Claimed to be fast-acting, it is said to penetrate to the germinative layer where new skin cells begin to develop.

This one-hour treatment commences with a thorough cleansing and toning of the skin, followed by a gentle peel to exfoliate dead skin cells. This is followed by the use of a special 'anti-wrinkle tracer' device which looks like a miniature roll-on deodorant. This is said to give each line of the face an in-depth massage with a regulated amount of biological concentrate to help lift and smooth facial furrows. Next, a special hydrating gel containing liposomes and DNA is massaged into the skin. Finally, a gauze mask impregnated with pure collagen is applied to the face on top of a second application of hydrating gel.

## Benefits and Claims
This treatment is claimed to purify the skin, progressively diminish wrinkles, lift, support and firm sagging facial contours, and leave the complexion soft, smooth and radiant. For maximum benefit, a course of two treatments per week for the first two weeks is recommended, followed by monthly treatments thereafter, or whenever the skin needs special attention.

## Results
Although it is difficult to assess whether this treatment can actually diminish wrinkles on a progressive basis, it certainly can improve the tone, texture and appearance of your skin.

## Value for Money?
A little pricey to be affordable on an on-going basis, but much

**AVERAGE PRICE**

ซ ซ ซ

depends on how much money you are prepared to invest in your efforts to hold back the years. Could be a good value-for-money preventive treatment on a quarter-yearly or six-monthly basis.

# NON-SURGICAL FACE-LIFTING TREATMENTS

Until very recently, the surgeon's scalpel was the only option open to those who could no longer bear to witness the unkind transformation wrought by time upon their face. Now, however, thanks to a number of recent advances in medical technology, as well as new innovations in the field of holistic therapy, a whole new ground-breaking range of non-invasive treatments, techniques and methods are flooding the face-lift market. Some are based on electro-stimulation; others are said to be wholly natural techniques. But the one thing all these new 'non-surgical face-lifting treatments and therapies have in common is that they all lay claim to being the ultimate alternative to the cosmetic surgeon's knife. The question is: do they work?

## *Acupressure*

Sometimes referred to as acupuncture without the needles, acupressure involves fingertip pressure on specific points located on the body, head and face. The principles behind this treatment are very similar to acupuncture in that the main objective is to restore the balance of natural energies that flow through the invisible system of channels known as meridian lines. By applying fingertip pressure to specific points on the meridians called *tsubos* it is possible to stimulate or reduce energy flow to areas where imbalances exist.

As interest in complementary therapies increases, more and more practitioners are becoming aware of the benefits to be gained from taking an holistic approach to treating their clients.

Nowadays most salons employ at least one therapist who is either knowledgeable in this area, or who has been trained to incorporate acupressure techniques in every facial treatment.

## Benefits and Claims

Acupressure is said to relieve stress, headaches and muscular pains that can cause tension in facial muscles. Its main beauty claim lies in its ability to help stimulate the lymphatic system to drain away toxins, speed up the metabolic rate and improve both blood and lymph circulation. Benefits are said to include increased hydration of facial skin , reduced puffiness, firmer neck and facial muscles – all of which are important factors in delaying the ageing process – and some reduction in fine lines and facial wrinkles.

## Results

People who have experienced this type of treatment claim a noticeable difference in the feel and look of their skin for several days afterwards. After trying – and enjoying – the treatment herself, my researcher did wonder whether the apparent effects resulted merely from an increase in blood circulation due to manipulation of skin tissue. If such was the case, she reasoned, then any simple home facial could produce a similar result at far less cost and inconvenience.

This supposition was countered by the therapist's observation that, whilst any facial treatment that helped improve circulation would undoubtedly have *some* effect on the skin, it is unlikely that customers could achieve this for themselves without proper knowledge and some training or practice in locating the specific *tsubo* points that stimulate lymphatic drainage.

## Value for Money?

Painless, relaxing and definitely a worthy 'stress-buster', this type of treatment rates fairly high in terms of the feel-good factor. Those with a bottomless purse may find that a fortnightly or monthly treatment pays a reasonable return so far as their looks are concerned. But if your choice of treatments is limited by the size of your beauty budget, it might be worth comparing this type of facial treatment with one or two others before committing yourself to anything more frequent than a seasonal session.

**AVERAGE PRICE**

Ʉ Ʉ

## Bio-therapeutic E2000

Promoted as 'the most technically advanced micro-current facial-toning treatment available today', this facial-toning machine uses computer controlled, galvanic microcurrents to gently tighten and strengthen the muscles of the face and neck.

Although there are a variety of other facial-toning machines currently being launched on to the market, the claims of Bio-Therapeutic E2000 to be the most advanced rests on the company's assertion that, because their model has dual-channel, duo-tipped probes, it not only creates a better up-lift but also covers a wider area in a shorter period of time. (It is interesting to note that, according to the distributor's promotional literature to the trade, this time-reducing factor also provides a considerable benefit to the salon, insofar as the less time a therapist spends on each individual treatment the bigger the overall profit margin. To be fair, however, this information ought not necessarily to detract from the efficacy of the treatment itself.)

Treatment sessions each take 45–60 minutes. A course of 10–18 at weekly intervals is recommended according to skin condition and age. In order to maintain the effects of the initial course, regular tone-up sessions every four to six weeks are advised.

After cleansing the face, both you and the therapist are connected to the machine to form an electrical circuit which will charge your bodies with a very small electrical current. With the aid of two hand-held devices that are wired up to the machine, each of which has a set of twin cotton-tipped probes attached, the therapist works slowly over each individual line and wrinkle to gently stimulate the underlying muscle tissue. The treatment is totally painless.

**AVERAGE PRICE**

Between ♉ ♉ and
♉ ♉ ♉ per treat-
ment
(some salons offer
discounts when a
course of treatment
is booked in
advance).

## Benefits and Claims

Tiny electrical impulses are said to reprogramme the muscles of the face and neck, to stimulate the skin's elasticity and improve blood circulation. An immediate result is claimed after just one session. Sagging muscles lift, wrinkles become smoother and the resulting improvement in skin tone is said to continue for at least 24 hours following treatment. A course is said to result in a healthy, more youthful appearance.

## Results

Publicity photographs that are claimed to be 'unretouched' show a marked improvement in the overall appearance of their two subjects. There was a perceptible lifting of the jowls of one 'guinea pig', and the deep nose-to-mouth grooves of another had all but disappeared. Sample treatments taken by testers on one half of their face showed a visible improvement in the shape and tone of the side treated, but the results were only temporary. Reports from other testers verify that this treatment can make a significant difference but precisely how much of a difference is impossible to predict in advance as this inevitably varies between each individual.

## Value for Money?

This depends on how many treatments are required to achieve any significant result, and its ultimate effects. Overall this could work out as quite an expensive form of face-lift, especially if you have to commit to maintenance treatments for life. However, for those whose looks have suffered due to recent stress or illness, this could provide a much-needed lift in every sense of the word.

## Joseph Corvo's Natural Face-lift

Popularly known as Joseph Corvo's Zone Therapy, the credit for the discovery of the principles underlying this treatment rightfully belongs – by Corvo's own admission – to Franz Henbach who first introduced Corvo to his findings more than 30 years ago. In the intervening period, having applied what he terms a 'thinking, systematic approach' to the subject, Corvo has perfected a series of exercises. When performed daily, they are claimed not only to create external and internal beauty, but also to help 'keep the face looking young, strong, handsome, or beautiful well into old age'.

The technique has gained a worldwide reputation and a clientele that allegedly includes royalty, film stars, top politicians and businessmen. The famous romantic novelist, Dame Barbara Cartland, has written a testimonial to Corvo's approach that literally overflows with effusive recommendations. All in all, Corvo has earned himself the reputation of being the world's most famous practitioner of this form of health and beauty treatment.

## Benefits and Claims

Says Corvo in his bestselling book, *Zone Therapy*, 'Science tells us that the body is an electromagnetic field, with electromagnetic currents coursing round it. Ten main invisible electrical currents run through the body in line with the toes and fingers. The area that each current covers is called a zone. The body is divided into equal parts with five zones on the left side and five on the right. All organs, glands and nervous systems fall into these zones.'

By massaging certain pressure points, Corvo claims it is possible to change the size and shape of the underlying muscles to improve the facial features. Chins can be made larger, rounder and stronger; the jawline firmer; facial lines can be filled out; and the complexion can be improved. Massaging key points on the face, says Corvo, helps free blockages in the nerve endings, stimulates muscle tissue and allows adequate supplies of blood, oxygen, protein and minerals to reach the face.

More importantly, he maintains, when these pressure points are massaged firmly enough, they will stimulate the body's electromagnetic fields to effect beneficial changes in areas other than the face. Thus, as your whole being responds to this treatment, health problems can be overcome, and a new feeling of elation and wellbeing will be achieved.

## Results

With Dame Barbara Cartland, at 93, as a walking-talking advertisement for this health and beauty treatment, one hardly dares question the efficacy of Joseph Corvo's techniques. But I suspended credulity long enough to make some investigations of my own. According to a number of testers who followed the treatment plan as outlined in Zone Therapy, it really did seem to have some effect, not only on the way they looked, but also on the way they felt.

## Value for Money?

'Start it at 17 as a preventative measure,' claims Corvo, 'and you will never need plastic surgery.' Doubtless, this promise comes a little late for many women. Whatever your age, however, it is still worth investing what is a fairly minimal sum in either the video or the book, as both can be said to represent pretty good value for money – provided that you do stick to the facial exercise regime they demonstrate.

In the meantime, although she would be starting it two years later than prescribed, I am tempted to recruit my 19-year-old daughter as a researcher in order to subject Corvo's promise (quoted above) to the ultimate test. If you have 25 years or so to spare, watch this space...

AVERAGE PRICE

Joseph Corvo's
Natural Facelift
*video (Warner Home
Video) – from* 🌷

Joseph Corvo's
Zone Therapy
*(Vermillion) – a little under* 🌷

## Flash Lifting

Flash Lifting is the name of a French biological face-firming product claimed to be 'the most advanced bio-technological discovery for reducing wrinkle occurrence and skin ageing'. Based on bovine serum, it contains pure placental extracts, amniotic liquid, elastin, and DNA and RNA isolated under strict standards of hygiene. Deep frozen at $-82°C$, this product comes in the form of either a dermal stick sealed in an isothermal cover which can be kept in your freezer at home, or as a concentrated serum for salon use. The serum is designed to be incorporated into a galvanic facial treatment. Alternatively, it can be applied for its skin-tightening and lifting effects at the end of a normal facial treatment.

The idea of using frozen embryo cells as an anti-ageing therapy is not new. Swiss clinics have been researching and experimenting with these for years. In essence the theory is that, as long as young cells are kept frozen from the moment of their extraction, they can share their DNA genetic information with older cells to help regenerate and prolong their life.

When using the product at home, the face must be thoroughly cleansed before it is applied. After removing Flash Lifting from the freezer, it should be warmed in your hand or a towel for several minutes (without actually being allowed to melt) and then applied in small circles over the entire facial area. The stick should be returned to the freezer immediately after use, and the rest of the liquid should be massaged into the face until it has been absorbed.

### Benefits and Claims
Flash Lifting is claimed to quicken the pace of cell regeneration, close the pores, hydrate and refine skin texture, accelerate the healing process in damaged areas, revitalise the skin's natural defences, and have an immediate tightening, smoothing effect on the skin.

### Results
It is easy to dismiss this product out of hand as being a wonderful new gimmick dreamed up by a desperate marketing man. After all, cell therapy is one thing, but does a product really have to be kept in a freezer in order to work its magic on ageing skin? There is a great deal of supportive evidence, however, to suggest that certain enzymes in placental extracts can indeed increase cell activity in the skin.

Apparently, the activity of enzymes can be measured by a

**AVERAGE PRICE**

Salon facial treat-
ment with concen-
trated serum
ʊ ʊ ʊ ʊ
(an initial course of
treatments at twice-
weekly intervals, is
recommended,
backed up by
twice-yearly cours-
es thereafter).

Flash Lifting dermal
stick ʊ ʊ ʊ ʊ ʊ
(lasts approximately
28 days).

process known as 'Warburg testing' which clearly demon-
strates that, when placental extracts are prepared at room
temperature, the degree of enzymatic (or Warburg) activity
is very high. Conversely, extracts subjected to any form of
heat-treatment are noted for the fact that enzyme activity is
nil. Moreover, according to one scientific report, placenta
extracts used in cosmetic preparations do seem to have the
ability to revitalise and regenerate the skin by stimulating the
metabolic rate of the cells, and accelerating the rate at which
dead skin cells are shed. Increasing the turnover rate of cell
production is known to help create an appearance of smoother,
firmer skin texture and a younger complexion.

Whether this product can actually lift wrinkles and lines,
however, is a debatable point. Certainly there is evidence to
suggest that lines and wrinkles can be made to *appear* less
noticeable, but this is believed mainly to be due to increased
moisture which is known to have a 'plumping-out' effect.

Testers who have tried the Flash Lifting stick at home for
a period of weeks have reported that their skin looks and feels
softer, smoother and firmer, and some have even noticed an
improvement in the appearance of open pores. On the whole,
however, none could claim any visible diminishing of lines and
wrinkles, although several reported that the treatment did
seem to make a dramatic difference to the tone and colour of
their skin, which appeared to be far more even after use.

## Value for Money?

Like most new wonder treatments, Flash Lifting has acquired
its fair share of devotees. At such a high price, however, you
would need to be blessed with a high disposable income, and/or
a fair degree of blind faith, to commit to either option in the
absence of any scientifically established evidence or conclusive proof that your money would be well spent.

## Eva Fraser's Facial Workout

Based on a systematic programme of facial exercises designed to slow down the ageing process, this technique is claimed to have worked wonders on its founder, Eva Fraser, who alleges to have learned the basic technique from a 76-year-old woman who had previously used it to great effect. According to Ms Fraser: 'Facial muscles are more complex because they are attached to the skin. Without exercise, the muscles slacken, and the skin droops with them, forming pouches, jowls, bags and wrinkles.'

Although private consultations and courses can be arranged with Ms Fraser, the techniques of this treatment have been made more widely accessible through the publication of a book and the release of a video. The video, which comes in two parts, is well-made and well-presented, and the exercises are clearly and concisely demonstrated. Part one consists of easy-to-follow demonstrations of exercises for specific problems such as crow's feet, scowl lines and double chins, and part two teaches a series of daily routines.

### Benefits and Claims

While Eva Fraser claims that her system is not to be regarded as the secret of eternal youth, she maintains that it is never too late to start working those facial muscles. Apparently, her exercises have even been successful on a woman of 84.

### Results

If Eva Fraser's face is a testament to the efficacy of her programme (at the age of 64 she has been practising what she now preaches for over 14 years), her approach would appear to work. Testers who have tried these exercises claim they make your face feel as warm, flushed and achey as your body does after it has been put through a strenuous work-out at the gym. According to Ms Fraser, provided that you spend five minutes on her exercises every other day you should begin to notice a difference after six weeks, with very real results

**AVERAGE PRICE**

Course of person-alised tuition with Ms Fraser – from
ᨺ ᨺ ᨺ ᨺ ᨺ ᨺ ᨺ

Eva Fraser's Facial Workout *video* (*Video Vision*) ᨺ ᨺ

Eva Fraser's Facial Workout book (Viking) ᨺ

becoming visible after twelve.

## Value for Money?

It is worth investing in the book or video. If you commit your-self to the treatment, and it works for you, you may consider it to be the best investment you have ever made. If you fail to keep it up, or the results are not quite what you expected, the cost is low enough to be easily written off.

## Rejuvanessence

Rejuvanessence is claimed to be a unique and highly effec-tive method of facial rejuvenation. Originally known as the Rosenberg Technique (after its Danish inventor, Stanley Rosen-berg), it is based on a system of exercises involving hands-on facial muscle-manipulation.

Having modified and improved upon her former mentor's technique, Margaretta Loughran is said to have first discov-ered Rosenberg's therapy when looking for a face-lift herself. After just one treatment, Swedish-born Margaretta claims to have been so impressed, she immediately abandoned her plans for cosmetic surgery. Looking at photographs of Margaretta's face prior to therapy, and seeing its results before you in the flesh, one cannot help but be convinced that Rejuvanessence offers the best evidence yet that some so-called 'alternative' face-lifts really do seem to achieve a visibly dramatic effect.

Like other holistic therapies, Rejuvanessence is founded on a series of deep facial massages. These are geared towards manipulating the 91 muscles in the face, neck and shoulders to free blockages caused in surrounding connective tissue by toxic build-up as a result of poor nutrition, smoking, alcohol, tiredness, pain and stress. Treatment consists of six one-hour sessions of light-fingered massage techniques. The aim is to free the connective tissue from the deeper layers of muscle and bone in order to create sufficient space for the muscles to relax and for the face to regain its former flexibility.

At an initial consultation, aspects of your diet and lifestyle are examined to find out what is contributing to your situation, and a snapshot is taken with an instant camera so that the results can be compared at the end of your course. Margaretta's fingers then deftly manipulate the muscle and tissue on one side of the face, shoulder and neck in a series of tiny tweaking movements. Before commencing on the other side of the face, she will offer you a mirror so that you can assess for yourself the results achieved so far. Not only does the 'treated' section feel tinglingly light and flexible, but you can actually see an improvement in terms of the tone, texture, roundness and glow of the skin on that side of the face.

The second treatment concentrates predominantly on the skull and forehead; the third on the nose and eye area; the fourth on the jaw and surrounding area; and the fifth on the 37 muscles in the neck. The sixth, and final, session utilises the technique of kinesiology. This involves a series of muscle-testing movements to reveal to what extent any weaknesses may exist in the body's inner organs and to uncover any undiscovered food allergies or sensitivities.

Food supplements may be advocated, and an-ongoing programme of general health and dietary modifications may also be recommended.

## Benefits and Claims

- Helps bring the facial muscles back to life again.
- Improves the complexion and the skin's elasticity.
- Reduces wrinkles.
- Lifts problem areas.
- Releases stress and tension gently, safely and effectively.
- A course of six treatments, followed by one top-up session quarterly, can help make a significant improvement to your facial appearance and delay further signs of ageing.

## Results
Having experimented with this treatment myself, I can attest

**AVERAGE PRICE**

Trial session 🌷 🌷 🌷

Recommended
course of six
treatments
🌷 🌷 🌷 🌷 🌷 🌷

Follow-up quarter-
yearly treatment
🌷 🌷 🌷

to the fact that it certainly seems to make you feel calm, relaxed and strangely energised at the same time, while the facial muscles do actually feel remarkably different. So far as its claim to lift lines and wrinkles is concerned, while the reported results of other testers' ranged from 'a slight lifting effect' to 'a marked improvement', the improvements to my own face were less apparent. To be fair, however, a number of people did make comments to the effect that I looked more 'relaxed and rested' than usual.

## Value for Money?

Difficult to assess. While Rejuvanessence is a great deal cheaper than cosmetic surgery (and a darn sight more pleasant, too) the cost of treatment is still significant enough to cause some concern to the less well-off should the final result not be quite as startling as one might have hoped for.

## Sarogenic Therapy

First developed in the United states, sarogenic therapy was initially designed specifically to help victims of Bell's Palsy (a debilitating condition that often results in one half of the face being paralysed) to recover mobility in the affected areas of the face. The treatment proved so successful that many patients clamoured to have the other half of their faces treated too. It is also claimed to be gaining popularity with athletes and sports teams as an effective, pain-relieving treatment for injuries.

Sarogenic therapy uses micro-amps of electricity that deliver a low-frequency pulse of energy to the muscles and underlying tissue of the face. An electrical circuit is set up between the client, the machine and the therapist, to allow the micro-current to be conducted through the therapist's hands directly to the client's skin. With moistened hands the therapist massages specific facial muscles in a series of precise movements. Some are gently smoothed out, stretched and lengthened; others are shortened as appropriate.

This stimulation is claimed to penetrate the protein enzymes within the individual cells of the muscles and create a feed-back to the nucleus that in turn reactivates the genetic life force within each cell. This process is alleged to stimulate blood circulation, to create a firming-up and toning action within the muscle fibres, to correct sagging muscles and increase the support provided to the surface layers of the skin. The therapy works at a deeper level first in order to develop the well-toned foundation necessary to support the more superficial muscles.

## Benefits and Claims

- Helps lift sagging jowls.
- Helps diminish smile and frown lines.
- Improves the skin's elasticity.
- Increases blood circulation to the face.
- Has a rectifying action on oily and acne-prone skin.
- Helps close the pores.

## Results

In order to demonstrate the remarkable effects of this treatment, the therapist treated only one half of my face. Although the results were not quite as startling as they have been with some clients, close inspection revealed a slight but perceptible difference in the positioning of my features, with the treated side appearing to be marginally 'higher' than the left half of my face.

Although I did not personally pursue a course of treatment, one of my testers did. Having observed the results very closely, I can verify that, on this particular individual, they are nothing short of impressive. After 18 sessions, the lines on her forehead have disappeared, the skin on her face has tightened, her jowls and jawline look tighter, and the grooves running down from her nose to the corners of her mouth look far less deeply-etched. Moreover, she is more than happy to commit to a monthly top-up treatment in order to maintain this effect.

**AVERAGE PRICE**

One-hour treatment session 🍷🍷🍷🍷 (a significant reduction on this price can often be obtained when booking a course of 15 or more weekly treatments).

In addition, I also interviewed a former victim of Bell's Palsy. She is so delighted with the way the affected side of face has responded to treatment that she is now considering a second course in the hope that it will enhance the appearance of the rest of her face.

## *Value for Money?*

Undeniably pricey. Based on the results I have personally witnessed, however, this could prove to be an equally effective, and undeniably safer, alternative to cosmetic surgery for the scalpel-shy. As for those who would never contemplate surgery, yet still cannot abide seeing the evidence of time's footprints upon their face, this certainly appears to be one treatment that might actually be well worth saving up for.

## *Warning*

Sarogenics is not recommended during pregnancy, or for anyone fitted with a pacemaker. Results are also likely to be less pronounced on clients below the age of 35.

# PERMANENT MAKE-UP

Said to be based on an adaptation of a centuries-old technique used by Chinese artists, permanent make-up can be used to correct the shape and colour of the eyebrows and lips. It is claimed to be particularly suitable for the following:

- People with thin or non-existent eyebrows, and those who would like a more prominent browline.
- People with poor eyesight who have difficulty in applying make-up.
- Athletes and sportswomen who do not want to use make-up.
- People with scars in their eyebrows, or who have undergone plastic surgery which has altered the position of the eyebrows.
- Women who are allergic to eyebrow pencils.
- Women with thin or poorly outlined lips.

• Alopecia sufferers and chemotherapy patients.

Permanent make-up can be applied in a single session which could take as little as 15 minutes for the eyebrows, or as long as an hour for the lips. Having carefully assessed your features, the therapist will select an outline according to the shape of your face. This will be marked with a pencil first to make sure you will be satisfied with the final outcome. Using a sterilised needle-tipped instrument attached to a small electrical device, a powdered mineral pigment dye is scratched into the surface of the skin in a series of ultra-fine brush-like strokes.

The marks are said to be lasting, but not irreversible. This means that, despite being termed 'permanent', the colour will eventually fade, as the pigments are only 'injected' into the surface of the skin (the epidermal layer) and do not penetrate the dermal layers which lie beneath. Unlike tattooing, the process does not draw blood.

According to my chief researcher, Sue, who volunteered to be a guinea pig for permanent eyebrow make up, the actual procedure can be quite painful. What started off as a mildly uncomfortable series of repeated 'scratching sensations' across the brow bone, soon turned into a teeth-gritting tenderness that brought tears to her eyes. In between drawing-in each individual 'hair', the therapist applied a soothing lotion designed to reduce redness or swelling.

At the end of the treatment, Sue was advised to purchase two products (a bottle of soothing eye lotion, and another containing a special soothing cream), and to bathe the area in the lotion and apply the cream to her brows twice a day. She was also warned that, as the pigment oxidises in the atmosphere, it would initially go 'darker' for two or three days, and then settle down to its 'natural' lighter colour three or four days after that.

A second visit, which is included in the overall cost of treatment, is required one month after treatment to check the colour and, if necessary, add a little extra.

AVERAGE PRICE
―――
Permanent make-up
treatment
ʊ ʊ ʊ ʊ ʊ

Soothing Eye Lotion
& Cream ʊ

## Benefits and Claims

'Darkens' and defines light-coloured or sparsely haired eyebrows. Also helps make thin lips look fuller and thicker.

## Results

Nothing short of impressive. Sue's eyebrows (which had previously been non-existent due to having been over-plucked in her youth) looked astoundingly natural and beautifully defined and shaped. Three months after treatment, she is still 'absolutely delighted', not only with the appearance of her eyebrows but also on several other counts, too: 'Unless you have spent half your life worrying about whether you have accidentally rubbed one eyebrow off, constantly having to ensure that you always have a brow pencil to hand, you cannot even begin to understand what a miraculous gift this treatment is for people like me' reports Sue.

The results of a 'permanent make-up' treatment can last between one and three years, depending on the condition of your skin. Oily skin, for example, exfoliates more rapidly than dry skin, so the results may not be as long-lasting as one might expect with a drier skin type.

## Value for Money?

Sue's evaluation says it all.

# REFLEXOLOGY

An ancient art of foot massage widely practised by the Egyptians, reflexology was rediscovered earlier this century by an American physician who found that pressing certain areas on the feet could make the face go numb. Reflexology is founded on similar principles to acupuncture in that both recognise the existence within the body of channels – or lines – of energy. Where reflexology differs from acupuncture, however, is that treatment is concentrated solely on specific areas of the feet that are said to be connected, via the channels of energy, with every organ in the body. When acid crystals, wastes and unused calcium form deposits on the delicate nerve endings of the feet, the body's energy flow is said to be impeded, and the connecting organ adversely affected. When a reflexologist massages and manipulates the feet, these deposits can be broken down, thereby causing the whole body, including the affected organ, to be revitalised and re-energised.

According to practitioners, every organ and gland depends for its survival upon the ability to relax and contract. When a reflexologist works on the feet, he or she will be dealing almost exclusively with autonomic (involuntary) reflexes and the autonomic nervous system (the pathways along which stimuli and impulses travel through the feet and body). By applying pressure to the reflex points on the feet a reflexologist can very quickly identify any organs that may be suffering stagnation or blockage. The degree of discomfort or tenderness felt by the patient is directly linked to the degree of tension within the associated organ. Massaging the point helps disperse the crystals, ease the pain and alleviate the problem.

## Benefits and Claims

In addition to being a useful diagnostic tool, reflexology is also claimed to be effective in treating almost any ailment or problem including asthma, arthritic conditions, backache, liver disorders, skin problems, menstruation difficulties, pain, stress, emotional and psychological problems, and even obesity. By harmonising the body's vital energy balance, every organ and system in the body benefits.

According to one reflexologist I interviewed, many physical problems have their roots in emotion. People who cannot cope with the effects of trauma, for example, often refuse to recognise their emotional pain; this becomes locked within, only to resurface in the guise of a physical symptom of tension elsewhere in the body. By treating the body, via the feet, a reflexologist can unlock the tension in the mind, thus allowing the emotions to flow freely again.

Although, like most forms of holistic therapy, reflexology

lays no claim to being a beauty treatment, any therapeutic benefits obtained from it on a physical, psychological and emotional level also have the potential to affect the appearance.

## Results

My visits to a reflexologist resulted in providing me with all the proof I needed that this form of treatment works. Not only did she identify correctly every single problem area in my body (most noticeably my neck and lower back), but she also gave me a chillingly accurate diagnosis both of my previous medical history *and* my personality traits.

For a week after the first treatment, my neck and back problems progressively worsened. Two days after the second treatment, however, the pain began to ease, and then disappeared altogether after the third. (Other testers have also reported experiencing a similar pattern in which their symptoms became worse before they began to experience an improvement.)

## Value for Money?

Apart from being wonderfully relaxing and energising, reflexology provides excellent value for money both as a remedial and a preventive treatment.

## Note

If you think you are far too ticklish to be able to relax while someone works on your feet, think again. Reflexologists seem to have a remarkable facility for 'desensitising' the feet.

---

**AVERAGE PRICE**

Per one-hour
session 𝐔 𝐔

---

# SCLEROTHERAPY

Sclerotherapy is the medical term for the treatment of broken (also known as 'thread') veins, slender capillaries that lie just beneath the surface of the skin. The walls of the capillaries have a certain elastic flexibility in that they dilate and contract in response to certain stimuli. Spicy foods, alcohol and heat can all cause the capillaries to expand temporarily. Occasionally, these tiny little blood vessels become so stretched that they lose their ability to contract to their normal size. This results in a permanently visible appearance of tiny red lines, or broken veins. If several capillaries are affected in a small area (such as the cheeks or the nose) they create a blotchy patch, or an appearance of 'ruddiness' in the complexion.

Some people simply have the kind of skin that is prone to broken veins. With others the cause is often due to such factors as poor circulation, excessive exposure to the sun and wind, a diet rich in spicy foods, or over-indulgence in alcohol, coffee and strong tea.

Sclerotherapy is a minor surgical procedure that involves injecting a sodium sulphate-based liquid through the epidermis into the capillaries. This causes them to shrink and fade. Each treatment session lasts 30–40 minutes. Depending on the number of capillaries, and the size of the area requiring treatment, it can take anything from three to six sessions for all the thread veins to disappear. In some cases there can be bruising which may last for up to three weeks.

## Benefits and Claims
Sclerotherapy can improve the complexion and the appearance of skin on other areas of the body (such as the legs) by removing most or all visible broken capillaries.

## Results
Remarkably successful. Moreover, the results can be permanent, provided that you eliminate the above-mentioned contributory factors. You should also be cautious about the sun, and avoid all forms of heat treatment such as saunas, steam treatments and very hot baths.

## Value for Money?
Very good. One tester felt this was a very small price to pay to get rid of her 'countrified complexion'.

| AVERAGE PRICE |
| :---: |
| Per treatment |
| ♉ ♉ |

# SAUNAS

The human body contains more than two million eccrine (or sweat) glands. Although these are distributed throughout the body, they are concentrated more highly in some areas than others – most noticeably the armpits, the palms of the hands and the soles of the feet. The body also contains a larger set of sweat glands, known as the apocrine glands. These are situated in the genital region and the area of the breasts, but do not develop until puberty.

Sweat glands have two main functions: they act as an excretory organ to remove waste-products from the body in the form of water and salts, and they also help regulate body temperature. On average, the body secretes 1–1.9 litres of sweat every 24 hours, most of which evaporates immediately.

Throughout the centuries sweating has been recognised and approved as a perfectly natural, healthy – and even desirable – bodily function. Nowadays, however, society has made such a virtue out of cleanliness, that we have come to view sweating as an undesirable and socially unacceptable activity. And while it is perfectly understandable – and even practical – for us to take extra measures in order to prevent us ruining our clothing, and possibly offending our friends and associates, the plain truth is that our over-reliance on heavy-duty antiperspirants and air conditioning is not healthy.

Too few of us sweat as much as we should. We are so concerned about cleansing our external appearance that we fail to use our body's own built-in purification process to keep our internal system clean. The more steps we take to avoid sweating in the normal way, the more essential it is that we make time to allow our body's own purification process to have full reign. The best way of achieving this is by subjecting ourselves to some form of heat treatment, such as a sauna.

Saunas are specifically designed to make the body sweat. Depending on the method of heating, and the degree of humidity achieved, a sauna can create a steam bath or a dry-heat bath, either one of which will encourage the body to respond to the heat by working extra hard to cool itself down. Saunas are like exercise – both put the body under similar stress. As your body works harder to throw off the heat, respiration increases and becomes heavier, the heartbeat and pulse quicken and grow stronger, and all the body's blood vessels dilate. As the body reacts internally to the stimulus of heat, perspiration breaks out.

Sweating causes fluid loss. Just one hour of sweating can result in a loss of around two litres of water. Moreover, with each teaspoon of fluid lost, the body will burn up around 3 calories, so in 10–15 minutes you can burn up an equivalent number of calories (100–250) as you would by walking one mile.

The usual guideline for using a sauna is to alternate one or two 10-minute sessions with a brief, cool shower. If you feel uncomfortable sooner, however, then you should immediately step out as there is no point in making a martyr of yourself. At the end of the final session, you should rub yourself down with a rough towel or loofah, moisturise your body and then lie down and relax for anything up to one hour.

Those who suffer from diabetes, hypertension or heart conditions should always seek medical advice before using a sauna.

## Benefits and Claims
Saunas can cause an immediate and often dramatic loss of weight through eliminating excess water from the tissues. In addition, they help detoxify the body, increase the circulation, draw out deep-seated grime and debris from the skin's pores, ease tension out of strained muscles, alleviate pain and menstrual cramping, and relax the body and the mind.

## Results
Apart from achieving all of the above, saunas can be wonderfully invigorating. However, most or all of the weight lost is likely to return as soon as you have a drink.

## Value for Money?
Excellent.

---

**AVERAGE PRICE**

Per session 💶
(free use of saunas and steam baths is usually included in membership of health and sports clubs).

# SHIATSU

A therapy of Japanese origin which has become increasingly popular over recent years, shiatsu is said to be an extremely precise and subtle method of diagnosis and treatment of minor ailments. Like acupuncture and reflexology, shiatsu works by stimulating the body's vital energy flow (termed 'chi' by the Chinese and 'ki' by the Japanese) in order to promote good health. With shiatsu, however, the therapist uses his thumbs, fingers, elbows, and even his knees and feet, to apply pressure and stretching to the meridian lines of energy. In the hands of a skilled therapist, shiatsu is said to revitalise or restore health by promoting the circulation of energy in the meridian lines, thus regulating the function of the organs, blood and body fluids, and increasing nourishment to the muscles and joints to aid flexibility and relaxation.

During a consultation, the therapist will take a detailed medical history and ask a great deal of questions. He will want to know all about your diet and lifestyle, what kind of exercise you take and how often, what job you do and what influences are at work in your life at that precise moment. These are designed to help the therapist gain a complete picture that will incorporate every aspect of your mental, emotional, physical and psychological state of being.

The Japanese are said to have perfected the art of abdominal diagnosis (which they term 'hara'), whereby the abdomen is palpated gently to determine the energetic quality and balance of the various internal organs. A shiatsu therapist will use both *hara* and pulse diagnosis to make an overall assessment of your health and to pinpoint any imbalances that might be disturbing your energy flow, or *ki*. When problems occur the *ki* will either be depleted ('kyo') or overactive ('jitsu').

During the actual treatment, the practitioner will work on the hundreds of points along the meridian lines called 'tsubos' in order to rebalance the 'yin' (negative) and 'yang' (positive) energy flow within the body.

## Benefits and Claims

According to Oriental therapists, the overt symptoms of illness are always preceded by an imbalance of *ki*. By rebalancing the body's vital flow of energy, shiatsu claims not only to prevent many diseases from manifesting, but also to help cure them once they have taken hold. Ailments that are said to respond well to shiatsu treatment include:

* headaches
* migraines
* respiratory illnesses including asthma
  and bronchitis
* sinus problems
* catarrh
* insomnia
* tension
* anxiety
* depression
* fatigue
* weakness
* digestive disorders
* bowel trouble
* menstrual pain
* circulatory problems
* rheumatic and arthritic complaints
* back trouble
* sciatica
* many sports strains and injuries

## Results

Although this is one of the few treatments that I have not personally tried, I have it on good authority that it is tremendously beneficial in a variety of ways. One tester claimed it helped cure her back problems, while another said she had suffered fewer asthma attacks since starting treatment. As with reflexology, it is apparently quite common to experience a variety of different reactions in response to treatment as the energy within the body shifts and balances.

## Value for Money?

Shiatsu appears to be a valid (and often remarkably success-ful) complementary treatment for many disorders. If you prefer the natural approach, then this will definitely provide good value for money.

AVERAGE PRICE

Per session

♉ ♉

## SOLAR THERAPY AND SUN BEDS

Phototherapy – the exposure of the body to the sun's ultra-violet (UV) rays – has long been recognised as a vital and integral part of treating a range of ailments. Despite being practised as a health treatment since ancient times, the ther-apeutic uses of solar therapy became more fully apparent only in the late 19th century when the Danish physician, Neils Ryberg Finsen, found that patients treated to regular doses of sunlight had a better recovery rate. Inspired by his discovery, Finsen invented the very first mechanical source of direct arti-ficial light (the first sun lamp). By no means perfect, Finsen's sun lamp nonetheless became accredited with successfully heal-ing the skin of smallpox victims and curing many cases of tuberculosis. This pioneering work won Finsen the Nobel prize for medicine in 1903.

While there has been much publicity in recent years about the dangers of over–exposing the body to the sun's harmful rays, there is no doubt that, providing it is taken in extremely carefully controlled doses, UV radiation from sunlight and artificial solaria can have a beneficial influence on the body. The sun emits a spectrum of electromagnetic rays, some of which are prevented from reaching the Earth's surface by the protective 'ozone' layer in the stratosphere. Of the total energy received at Earth level, around 56 per cent is infra–red, and approximately 39 per cent what is known as 'visible light', both of which penetrate quite deeply into the body. The remaining 5 per cent of energy received on Earth is in the form of UV radiation. And while too much infra–red light can be bad for us, it is UV radiation, in particular, which can have the most serious consequences for our skin.

UV rays come in three types: UV-A, UV-B, and UV-C. The latter are of little concern as they tend to be absorbed by the ozone layer. UV-B rays are the ones that make us burn. The reason for this is that, although they only make up about 2 per cent of the UV spectrum, they are mostly absorbed just above the dermis. And whilst UV-A rays, which are able to penetrate very deeply into the dermis and beyond, are predominantly responsible for providing us with a tan, these particular rays also have the most sinister long-term effects.

When you expose your body to the sun, a physiological reaction takes place. The UV rays absorbed by the body trigger off a protective mechanism by stimulating the production of brown pigments (melanin) which cause the skin to redden and darken. If exposure continues for any length of time, the UV-B rays will then stimulate the melanocytes (the cells that produce melanin) to step up their productivity rate. The fact that it can take between two to five days for the melanocytes to produce sufficient melanin to create a protective tan is the main reason why we should always be especially vigilant about over-exposing ourselves to the sun's rays during the early days of our holiday. Too much sun, too soon, is likely to result in severe burning.

Apart from giving us an opportunity to acquire a year-round tan, sun beds and solaria can be useful in providing us with a range of additional benefits. It is essential, however, that they are used sensibly, safely, and with the utmost caution.

## Benefits and Claims

Everyone feels better with a suntan. Apart from making us look slimmer, fitter, healthier and younger, a suntan can do wonders for our self-confidence.

According to recent research, concentrated bursts of lengthy sunbathing over a short period of time (as usually happens when we are on holiday) is far more dangerous in the long term than shorter, more frequent periods of regular, controlled exposure. There is also the risk of painful burns and scarring.

Psychologically, a suntan is implicitly associated with affluence, attractiveness, desirability and success. Physiologically, UV-B rays are predominantly responsible for causing the synthesis of Vitamin D in the skin. Sunbeds and solaria are also useful in helping to treat certain conditions, such as skin problems and seasonal affective disorder (SAD).

SAD is a form of depression that often affects victims in the autumn and disappears in spring. Characteristic symptoms include inexplicable bouts of depression (often accompanied by sleep-disturbance), over-eating, decreased physical activity and problems with personal relationships. Early research indicates that a deficiency of light can adversely affect the metabolic and endocrine system in susceptible individuals. UV light from solaria, and other sources, is alleged to have effected a number of 'cures'.

### Results

All forms of solaria and sun-bed treatments will accelerate a tan, but there are a number of risks attached. It has been estimated that artificial UV light emits 10 times more radiation than you would receive from the sun when it is at its most powerful, such as at noon in summertime. Moreover, its effects are cumulative. This means that the more you use them, the greater the risk of developing wrinkles, discoloured patches and cancer in later life. UV rays also dehydrate the hair, and leach it of its natural protective oils. Fair-skinned people and those with red hair are most at risk.

If you must use a solarium, always do so with the utmost caution. Innovations are taking place all the time, and most manufacturers are becoming increasingly conscious of the need to provide in-built safeguards in order to minimise the potentially damaging effects of UV rays. Nevertheless, you should be extremely vigilant about obeying the manufacturer's recommended precautions.

Under no circumstances should you use a sun bed in any of

the following instances:

- During a period of antibiotic treatment, and for up to 7 days afterwards.
- During pregnancy.
- If you have ever had any form of radiation treatment.
- Whilst taking the contraceptive pill, as this could result in uneven colouring.
- If you have a heart condition, a pace-maker, epilepsy or have had organ-transplant surgery.
- If you suffer from cataracts, moles, migraines, diabetes, urinary problems or kidney disorders.

Moreover, not only is it advisable to remove every trace of make-up, perfume and deodorant from your skin (these can cause burning and irritation), but you should never use a sunbed without wearing protective goggles, as UV light can cause permanent eye damage if it is allowed to burn the cornea.

## Value for Money?

If you cannot conceive of appearing in public without a tan, then you would probably regard this form of treatment as good value for money. Given the very real dangers linked to over-exposure to both the sun, and all forms of solaria and sun beds, however, I cannot stress highly enough that anyone considering this form of treatment should balance their immediate desire for a tan against the long-terms risks associated with the process of acquiring it. When assessed realistically, any of the alleged benefits that are said to accrue from possessing a tan (and to my mind these have been proved to be so minimal as to be immediately discountable) are far outweighed by the long-term hazards to our physical health and well-being.

# TONING TABLES

When toning tables first appeared on the market, they were welcomed everywhere as the 'slimmer's salvation'. Promoted as the most sophisticated, and absolutely effortless inch-loss system ever launched, women the world over flocked to their local salons, desperate to discover for themselves what it must be like to realise their long-held dream of 'simply being allowed to lie there while a machine whittled away every excess inch'.

Like most new slimming products, toning tables have had their 10-minute burst of fame and acclaim. And although they have attracted their (largely unfair) share of bad publicity (mainly due to the few salon owners who lacked sufficient training and knowledge to teach clients their proper use), they now appear to have established for themselves a natural niche in the trimming-and-slimming treatment market.

A toning table 'treatment' usually takes around one hour. During this time you will complete a 'circuit' of isometric-type exercises using anything between five and ten different tables, each one designed to stretch, exercise and tone a different set of muscles. All toning tables have movable sections which, when switched on, will lift the legs, turn the ankles, or move a variety of different parts. They *do not* 'do' the exercises for you, as that would be totally pointless. What they can do is provide a little support for the part of the body being moved and to give your muscles something to 'resist' against. In giving the entire body a workout, they can help improve overall flexibility without overworking the muscles.

## Benefits and Claims

Claims range from the ridiculous, such as 'incredible inch-loss with absolutely no effort involved', to the reasonable, such as 'reduces measurements by helping to tone and tighten each individual muscle group'. Just 10 minutes on some machines is said to be equivalent to anything from a two-mile walk or 90 sit-ups to 900 back–kicks (how *do* they know?)

Toning tables are claimed to help stimulate the circulation

of blood and lymph, increase joint flexibility and mobility, and aid the body's eliminatory process. They also are said to be ideal for people with physical limitations, such as those who suffer from arthritis or back pain, as well as the elderly.

### Results

Far from being effortless, toning tables are *not* an easy option – if you want to see results, you have to be prepared to work hard. Do not expect miracles, as it can often take five to six sessions before any real inch loss can be measured. Best results have been found when people exercise a minimum of three times a week for at least four to five weeks. Like many other 'toning' treatments, however, the moment you stop, back come the inches.

### Value for Money?

Yes, if you are prepared to work at it, and to keep on working at it with a maintenance programme. Otherwise, save your money.

| AVERAGE PRICE |
| :---: |
| Per session – from |
| ♉ |
| (discounts are offered on the single-session price if you are prepared to book up a course). |

## VACUSAGE

A form of electrical massage treatment, Vacusage can be used on the face to improve the complexion and reduce puffiness by encouraging lymphatic drainage, and also on the body as an aid-to-slimming treatment. Most treatment sessions last for 15–30 minutes.

The Vacusage equipment consists of an electrical machine with a motor-driven vacuum pump and one or more leads with clear-plastic suction cups attached. When the machine is switched on, a partial vacuum is created beneath the cups. As the therapist glides the cups slowly and gently along the path of the lymph vessels, the skin will 'suck up' into the cups. The object of the exercise is to increase the rate of lymph flow and to convey softened fat cells in the lymph to the nearest lymph node where the fat and toxins will be released.

Vacusage is not recommended for clients with heart problems, varicose veins, pacemakers or metal plates, or indeed for anyone who may be pregnant or recovering from recent surgery.

### Benefits and Claims

Vacusage claims to help slimming by breaking down and dispersing softened fat, and to help tighten up saggy skin.

### Results

Vacusage works best on areas of excessive soft fat. It is most effective when used either as a firming aid after severe weight loss, or in conjunction with other slimming treatments and dieting.

### Value for Money?

Yes, if you have a problem with poor circulation and lymph drainage, and/or if you are determined to have a serious blitz on your body fat.

## VIBROSAUN

Vibrosaun is a revolutionary body-conditioning system that is proving especially popular with sports professionals for whom weight is a crucial issue, such as jockeys and boxers. An Australian invention, Vibrosaun is claimed to be the result of a long and intensive study by a team of highly qualified people including a medical practitioner, a chiropractor, an osteopath, a physiotherapist and a design engineer. Their prime intention is said to have been to create a simple, economical and universal machine that would, as near as possible, simulate exercise without putting stress on the body.

Designed to be controlled from within by the client, the Vibrosaun machine looks like a more comfortable version of a toning table with a large lid on top. It functions as a combined sauna and vibrating massage machine: the vibration stimulates

| AVERAGE PRICE |
| :---: |
| Per 30-minute session 🌷 |

and relaxes the muscles, while the dry heat dilates the blood vessels and increases the metabolism, heart and pulse rate. This in turn is said to increase the blood flow and stimulate metabolic consumption of oxygen to create energy and burn carbohydrates, protein and fat cells, whilst accelerating kidney function and the removal of lactic acid and blood wastes.

Best of all, because your head is not enclosed, and the machine also has a fan built into the headrest to ensure you are constantly wafted with cool, fresh air, not only is there no feeling of claustrophobia or suffocating heat, but your hair stays totally dry and 'unmessed'.

## Benefits and Claims

The Vibrosaun concept is claimed to offer innumerable benefits wrapped up in one treatment. The combination of dry-heat sauna and massage is claimed to help relieve muscular aches and pains, to aid lymphatic drainage and the detoxification process, to help slimming and weight control, increase blood circulation, simulate exercise, promote perspiration, and also to provide deep stress and relaxation therapy.

As this machine is multifunctional, it can be used in conjunction with a variety of therapeutic treatments including aromatherapy massage, body wraps and cellulite therapies. Moreover, it is said to be especially beneficial in the treatment of sports injuries, and in alleviating arthritic and rheumatic pain.

## Results

Excellent! This is an incredible invention that not only feels great, but offers all the therapeutic benefits of several different treatments wrapped up in one. This is the nearest thing to an almost miraculous and effortless slimming, toning and detoxifying treatment I have ever come across. It is truly so effortless that you can even drift off to sleep as your body is lulled into relaxation by the combined effects of gentle waves of warm, dry heat, rhythmic movement and soothing music. It is much more comfortable than a sauna, and because you can control the temperature yourself, you only get as much heat as you can personally take. It is also the perfect solution for shy people who would rather not expose their bodies to all and sundry.

## Value for Money?

Considering the amount of money you can save by combining several different treatments in one, this is excellent value for money.

---

**AVERAGE PRICE**

Single 25–30 minute session 🌷

Combined with aromatherapy or body-wrap treatment 🌷🌷

PART TWO

# *Health Resorts*

I N THE 1940S AND 1950S, the mere mention of a health resort, (or 'fat farm' as they were more popularly known) would have been enough to fill the average person with alarm. The prospect of being confined to an establishment where one would be subjected to a Spartan diet and an exhausting regime of punishing exercise was far too uncomfortable a proposition to warrant being anyone's idea of recreation. The health resorts of the past rightly deserved their reputation for being a form of purgatory – nightmare institutions to be endured exclusively, and solely in the spirit of penance, by those desperately seeking absolution for their dietary misdeeds.

Today's health resorts have come a long way over the last decade or two. In striving to cast off their erstwhile negative image, they have successfully managed to establish themselves as a group of inviting oases offering the perfect antidote to the many pressures and problems of modern life. And while this panacea is available only at a price, there is a growing army of people, from virtually all walks of life, who now regard their regular trips to such places as providing not so much an opportunity for self-indulgence, but a prescription for a long and healthy life.

The main attraction of the larger, more luxurious health resorts lies in the fact that they offer an unprecedented opportunity for self-gratification. Amid surroundings of incredible luxury, you can hone and tone your body to new levels of fitness in a superbly equipped gym; gain instruction in virtually any new form of sport; or indulge your passion for golf, horse riding, tennis or just about any other physical activity that takes your whim.

Alternatively, you can opt for the more seductive route. This simply involves allowing the days to merge effortlessly and idly into each other as you drift through a series of treatment rooms. A battery of beauty therapists will massage, pamper and cosset your face and body until every lump, bump, wrinkle and tension-traced line is magically smoothed away. If relaxation is your goal, I can personally testify that the latter route will leave you so relaxed you will be almost comatose – at the end of one idyllic week at such an establishment it took me several days to recall my own telephone number!

Furthermore, the chances of being confronted by the offensive sight of a lone lettuce leaf or a glass of lemon juice are virtually nil. With some of the best chefs in the business in charge of the menus, the cuisine often spans the gamut from *nouvelle* to *haute*, and the only restrictions that are likely to apply to the size of your plate are those governed by the dictates of your own appetite.

And then there are the treatments – the icing on the cake of every hedonist's dreams! They are designed to pander to every conceivable desire, need or whim, from high-tech beautifying treatments to holistic therapies aimed at treating, harmonising and unifying every aspect of your mind, body, spirit and soul. The allure of all modern health resorts, regardless of each one's size or individual philosophy, is that they all but guarantee to make a glowing, youthful, stress-free silk purse out of any old sow's ear.

The fact is, there are some temptations in life that are virtually irresistible, and the modern health resort is definitely one of these. But be warned – all this luxury, pampering and self-indulgence does not come cheap!

While I have tried to provide a fair guide to a reasonable number of health resorts in order to help narrow down your choice, the following list is by no means conclusive. Apart from which, certain details, prices, activities and facilities are inevitably subject to change. Before committing yourself, it would therefore be a wise precaution to conduct a little research of your own by sending off for any brochures, and following this up with a telephone call if any questions remain unanswered.

Some resorts offer special weekend or short-break programmes at discounted rates. If you can be flexible in your arrangements, it is worth checking these out as you may be able to make a significant saving simply by switching your planned vacation to another date.

Facilities, services and any special packages of treatment inclusive in the overall price can vary quite considerably between resorts. Beauty treatments are usually optional and expensive extras, so if you have your heart set on trying a number of specific therapies and treatments outlined in the brochure, make sure you know precisely how much these are likely to add to the cost of your stay *before* you book. It is all too easy to succumb to temptation at a preliminary consultation session, especially when payment is deferred until the end of your stay. Deciding in advance how many extras you can afford, and sticking to your budget, can save embarrassment and regret when it comes to settling your final bill.

While it is always nicer and more comfortable to share any new experience with a friend, you need not feel nervous about visiting a health resort alone if you cannot find anyone to join you. Unlike many hotels, most health resorts are very conscientious about putting lone visitors at ease. Some put aside a special table in their restaurants where a resident host or hostess takes care of any introductions and makes sure the conversation flows.

Although the services and facilities provided as part of the overall package tend to vary, these generally include the following:

- Accommodation and all meals, plus any fruit juices, tea or coffee (these are usually available throughout the day, but any wine ordered with your meals will be charged to your bill).
- Medical consultation with a qualified nurse or doctor, at which time your blood pressure and full medical history will be taken (a more detailed medical examination is often available at additional cost).
- Consultation with a dietician or nutritionist (but clients are not forced to diet against their will).
- Use of all fitness and sports facilities, such as the gymnasium, pool, exercise classes, tennis courts and bicycles.
- Entertainments, such as television, videos, lectures or talks given by visiting experts, art and craft instruction/classes, and other recreational facilities such as snooker and chess.

A free central reservations and advisory service providing advice on health hydros and spas in Britain has been set up by Healthy Venues, 45 Armorial Road, Coventry CV3 6GH, telephone (0203) 690300.

## HEALTH RESORTS IN BRITAIN

Please note that, unless otherwise stated, prices given are for a single occupancy of a standard room.

CEDAR FALLS HEALTH FARM
*Bishops Lydeard, Taunton, Somerset TA4 3HR*
*Telephone: (0823) 433233*
Cedar Falls is set in 44 acres of beautiful landscaped gardens and grounds, complete with trout-fishing lake, at the foot of the Quantock Hills in rural Somerset. It is neither as grand, nor as expensive, as some of the larger, more up-market British health resorts.

The building, which resembles a country manor-house hotel, is an award-winning conversion of an 18th-century red sandstone mansion of some historical interest. The atmosphere is cosy and reassuring, attracting a mixed clientele including affluent businessmen, stressed-out executives, middle-managers, media personalities, minor celebrities, career women and housewives.

Free fitness and sporting facilities include:
- 18-hole golf course
- croquet
- exercise room
- heated indoor and outdoor swimming pools
- horse-riding and squash (can be arranged at local establishments at additional cost)
- outdoor badminton
- tennis courts
- trim track and bicycles

- trout-fishing lake
- whirlpool

Inclusive in the tariff:
Three treatments daily from a list including steam or sauna, massage, solarium, aromatherapy and peat bath.

Optional extras include:
- acupuncture
- aromatherapy
- beauty-salon treatments
- body wraps
- cranial sacrial therapy (manipulation of the cranium)
- facials (including collagen facial treatments)
- hypnotherapy
- Ionithermie
- iridology
- mud packs
- osteopathy
- reflexology
- shiatsu
- Slendertone
- stress-management course

<table>
<tr><td>AVERAGE PRICE</td></tr>
<tr><td>Per night<br>♨ ♨ ♨ ♨<br>(minimum stay 3 nights).</td></tr>
</table>

CHAMPNEYS AT TRING
*Wiggington, Tring, Herts HP23 6HY*
*Telephone: (0442) 863351*
Widely regarded as the Rolls Royce of British health resorts, Champneys has a reputation for attracting a clientele drawn from the ranks of the rich, the famous and the titled. Rumours abound to the effect that the atmosphere at Champneys is intimidating, haughty and competitive. This is said to be mainly due to a hardcore contingent of female regulars whose main preoccupation is vying to outdo one another with their showy displays of jewellery and inexhaustible supply of designer bathrobes and dressing gowns.

These rumours are totally without foundation. Having stayed at Champneys myself, I can personally attest to the fact that, while the atmosphere is genuinely luxurious, and every facility of the highest professional standard, there is little about this establishment (including the attitude of its clientele) that should make the average working person feel in the least bit uncomfortable or out of place. The only thing that might make the lesser-monied feel like a poor relation – and the same also could be said to apply to many other health resorts – is the fact that you might not be able to indulge yourself in as many beauty treatments as you would like due to the relatively high costs involved.

The only other factor that may have a bearing on allegations about the 'anti-social' attitude of some guests is that around 50 per cent of Champney's weekend clientele usually consists of couples intent on relaxing and rediscovering the joys of togetherness. In my experience, if you are prepared to overcome your own shyness in the first instance, and put yourself out to be friendly in the second, others will respond accordingly.

Free sporting, fitness and recreational facilities include:
- bicycles
- dance studio
- games room
- large indoor swimming pool
- leisure arts and craft centre
- putting green
- squash courts (2)
- tennis courts
- volleyball
- well-equipped gymnasium

Private sports tuition can be arranged at extra cost, as can horse riding and golf at nearby establishments.

Free activities programme includes:
- advice on exercise and nutrition

- aerobics, stretch and step classes
- beauty demonstrations
- beginners' squash
- body-conditioning circuits
- guided walks
- hydro fitness
- jazz-dance sessions
- juggling
- professional art tuition
- relaxation
- series of talks on such topics as 'NLP', 'Self-esteem and Self-development', 'Positive Thinking' and 'The Alexander Technique'.
- swimming lessons
- t'ai chi chu'an
- yoga

Inclusive in the tariff:
Two treatments daily (except on Sundays and day of arrival) including a massage (underwater, full-body or neck and shoulders), plus a heat treatment (sauna and plunge, spa bath or steam).

Optional extras include:
- aromatherapy
- Aromazone therapy (lymphatic massage)
- beauty-salon treatments (waxing, bleaching, eyelash and eyebrow tinting, manicures, pedicures, professional make-ups, hairdressing)
- body wraps
- bust and body treatments
- reflexology
- special facial, neck, and eye treatments
- sun beds and tanning treatments
- Thai Massage
- Vibro massage with G5

Medical and paramedical services available at extra cost include:

- acupuncture
- back-care course
- blood tests
- chiropody
- cholesterol testing
- computerised fitness assessment (comprising body-fat, lung-function and stamina tests)
- general medical consultation
- Medi-check screening for men and women
- nutritional analysis
- orthopaedic consultations
- osteopathy
- physiotherapy
- stop-smoking programme
- well-woman consultations (including cervical smear, mammography, breast examination)

---

**AVERAGE PRICE**

**Per night**

🌷 🌷 🌷 🌷 🌷

(minimum stay two nights).

**Per week – from**

🌷 🌷 🌷 🌷 🌷 🌷 🌷
🌷 🌷 🌷

---

FOREST MERE HEALTH HYDRO
*Liphook, Hampshire GU30 7JQ*
*Telephone: (0428) 722051*
Set in 150 acres of tranquil woodland with lawns and a lake, Forest Mere's ambience is one of relaxed, comfortable elegance. One of the main attractions is its reputation for providing the little extra touches of cosseting and comfort that appeal especially to its worn-out, work-weary clientele, which comprises all kinds of people from every stratum of society. The staff, many of whom have been with the resort for years (always a very good sign) are said to be exceptionally warm, friendly, caring and even motherly in their ministrations; an approach that is obviously relished by the clientele, if the number returning for several 'winding-down' sessions each year is anything to go by.

In addition to the usual three wholesome meals per day, the

provision of afternoon tea complete with cakes (carefully calorie-counted in order not to tip anyone's dieting scales the wrong way) is an unusual and very popular additional touch.

Free sporting, fitness and recreational facilities include:
- bicycles
- billiards
- boating
- body toning to music
- films
- gymnasium
- heated pool
- hydrotherapy
- keep fit
- lectures
- light classical piano recital
- snooker
- table tennis
- tennis
- walking and jogging trail
- yoga

Golf and horse riding can be arranged locally at extra cost.

Inclusive in the tariff:
- consultations
- massage
- osteopathy
- sauna
- steam cabinet
- underwater massage

Optional extras:
- aromatherapy
- beauty and hair treatments
- body wraps
- chiropody
- colour analysis

- dietary therapy
- hypnotherapy
- manicure
- pedicure
- physiotherapy
- slimming treatments
- solaria

**AVERAGE PRICE**

Overall cost of a
minimum three-
night stay

ᵾ ᵾ ᵾ ᵾ ᵾ ᵾ ᵾ

## GRAYSHOTT HALL HEALTH AND FITNESS RESORT
*Headley Road, Grayshott, nr. Hindhead, Surrey GU26 6JJ*
*Telephone: (0428) 604332*

Grayshott Hall is set in 47 acres of landscaped grounds, which are surrounded by extensive countryside protected by the National Trust. A grand Victorian mansion, it owns the distinction of having being the former country retreat of one of Britain's best-loved poets, Sir Alfred Lord Tennyson. A popular retreat for many of Britain's theatrical and television stars, the atmosphere at Grayshott is best summed up as being peaceful, homely and very English.

Free sporting, fitness and recreational facilities include:
- 9-hole golf course (par 3)
- badminton
- bicycles
- billiard room
- cardiovascular fitness training
- circuit training
- croquet
- exercise studio
- gymnasium with hydra fitness equipment
- Hatha yoga
- heated indoor pool and spa bath
- low-impact aerobics
- outdoor tennis court
- putting green
- rebounder classes

Use of the new indoor two-court tennis centre is available at an extra charge.

Inclusive in the tariff:
Two treatments daily comprising massage (excluding day of arrival), and choice of heat treatment, such as sauna, steam cabinet or steam room.

Optional extras:
• aromatherapy
• Aromazone treatment
• beauty and hair-salon treatments (including specialist facials, hair and scalp treatments, manicures, pedicures)
• Blitz high-pressure water-jet treatments
• body wraps
• chiropody
• cholesterol screening
• energy-balancing treatment
• exercise training
• fitness assessments
• floatation-room treatments
• full medical screenings (including ECG, X-ray and blood analysis tests)
• holistic massage
• hydrotherapy baths
• individual golf lessons
• lifestyle counselling
• physiotherapy
• reflexology
• stop-smoking hypnotherapy
• swimming and tennis coaching
• t'ai chi massage

> **AVERAGE PRICE**
> ___
> **Per night**
> ♨ ♨ ♨ ♨ ♨ ♨
> (Recommended minimum stay four nights. Although guests can stay for shorter periods, special promotional offers of a complimentary fourth night are often used to encourage guests to stay for the recommended minimum period.)

HENLOW GRANGE HEALTH FARM
*The Grange, Henlow, Bedfordshire SG16 6DB*
*Telephone: (0462) 811111*

Housed in an impressive Georgian mansion set in acres of picturesque riverside parkland, this establishment places a considerable emphasis on exercise and sport. This is reflected in the number of leading international athletes, sports stars and fitness personalities whose faces are regularly seen at Henlow Grange (and also at its sister establishment – Springs Hydro in Leicestershire), not only as guests enjoying a break, but also as visiting instructors invited as part of the resort's special programme of master classes.

Free sporting, fitness and recreational facilities include:
- aquaerobics
- bicycles
- boating
- croquet
- dance classes
- floatation room
- floodlit tennis court
- gymnasium
- hydrotherapy bath
- indoor heated pool
- jazz dance
- step aerobics
- volleyball
- whirlpool
- yoga

Private swimming lessons and tennis coaching are available at extra charge. Horse-riding, badminton and golf can be arranged locally at additional cost.

Inclusive in the tariff:
Three treatments daily comprising a full-body or neck-and-shoulder massage, facial, sauna or Turkish bath.

Optional extras:
- aromamassage
- aromatherapy
- aromatherapy with reflex diagnosis
- beauty-salon and hair treatments
- bust-firming
- cellulite treatment
- facial treatments
- faradic muscle toning
- Finnish sauna and swim
- G5 vibro massage
- infra–red treatment
- manicures
- pedicures
- personal body alignment
- personal training and fitness assessment
- physiotherapy
- remedial massage
- seaweed baths
- slimming/firming treatments
- Swedish body massage
- toning tables
- vacuum suction
- yoga instruction (individual)

---

**AVERAGE PRICE**

Per night
ɰ ɰ ɰ ɰ ɰ

Per week
ɰ ɰ ɰ ɰ ɰ ɰ ɰ
ɰ ɰ ɰ

---

INGLEWOOD HEALTH HYDRO
*Kintbury, nr. Newbury, Berkshire RG15 OSW*
*Telephone: (0488) 682022*
Mentioned in the Domesday Book, Inglewood was one of the great houses of the Knights Templar during the Crusade of 1108, and later became a Royal Falconry during the reign of Henry VIII. Set in 50 acres of beautiful countryside on the edge of the Berkshire Downs, amidst a clutch of famous stables, studs and horse-training establishments, Inglewood has an atmosphere that combines the unadulterated luxury of stately-home grandeur with the informal friendliness and comfort of

a family-run country house hotel.

Inglewood has been described as the 'Marks and Spencer of health farms' because it provides a good quality service, without frills, at a reasonable price. Its clientele includes an eclectic mix of famous names of stage and screen, Arabian royalty, up-and-coming pop stars, business tycoons, executives, affluent housewives and career types. The emphasis is on rest, relaxation, tranquillity, good nutrition and optimum health. Because of its close association with the famous Norland Nannies training school a few short miles away (where babies and toddlers can be looked after during their parent's stay) Inglewood also attracts a number of better-off young mums seeking to regain their health and figures after childbirth.

Free sporting, fitness and recreational facilities include:
- bicycles
- clock golf
- croquet
- cycling
- evening talks and entertainments
- exercise, dance and stop-smoking classes
- games room with billiards, snooker, and table tennis
- gymnasium
- indoor swimming pool and jacuzzi
- jogging
- tennis
- yoga

Golf, squash, fishing, barge trips, horse-riding, and clay-pigeon shooting can be arranged locally at extra charge.

Inclusive in the tariff:
Four treatments daily (except Sundays when no treatments are given, and on midweek arrival and departure days when two treatments are available). These comprise one heat treatment (such as sauna, steam room, steam cabinet, peat bath or aroma-oil bath), and three body treatments which may be selected from G5, massage, Slendertone, osteopathy and

physiotherapy.

Optional extras:
* aromatherapy
* beauty-salon and hair treatments (including facials; manicure; moor, mud and wax baths)
* faradism
* G5
* massage
* peat bath
* pedicure
* radiant heat
* reflexology
* sauna
* short-wave diathermy
* Slendertone
* solarium
* specialist face and body treatments
* swimming lessons
* tennis coaching
* therapeutic inhalation

**AVERAGE PRICE**

**Per three-day minimum stay**

**Per week**

## THE LORRENS HEALTH HYDRO (LADIES ONLY)

*Cary Park, Babbacombe, Torquay TQ1 3NN*
*Telephone: (0803) 323740*

One of the few establishments catering exclusively for women, The Lorrens is on a far smaller scale than most health resorts. Far from detracting from its appeal, however, the snug, informal, intimate atmosphere and concentration on personal attention attracts all kind of women, from young to middle-aged, and from housewives to executives. The Lorrens offers them an opportunity to escape the pressures of their lives, lose weight, get fit and embark on a whole new life-enhancing regime. This is reflected by the fact that The Lorrens operates a no-smoking policy.

Set in a large house nestling between a beautiful park and

public gardens in the 'English Riviera' resort of Babbacombe, the emphasis at The Lorrens is on providing a healthy, well-balanced detoxification diet, and a programme of individually tailored exercise treatments to help clients shed weight and get fit. A popular speciality is the Slimaway programme. Lasting five or seven days, it incorporates a comprehensive range of treatments and activities (included in the price) specifically designed to achieve the best possible results.

If size, luxury and variety of facilities are any criteria by which to judge a health resort, The Lorrens cannot even begin to compete with the bigger establishments. But when it comes to price, professionalism, personal attention, success ratio and sheer value for money, it is an exceptionally worthy competitor by anyone's standards.

Free sporting, fitness and recreational facilities include:
• circuit training
• dance studio
• eucalyptus steam room
• gymnasium with cardio-vascular equipment and exercise studio
• jacuzzi
• low-and high-impact aerobics
• rebound training
• Step Reebok
• Viking pine sauna

Inclusive in the tariff:
Personal health and fitness assessment with computerised Positive Health Profile, plus 6 treatments daily from a range including sauna, G5, faradic treatment, anti-stress massage, steam treatment, vacuum suction, Sixtus footcare treatment and whole-body massage.

Optional extras:
• aromatherapy
• beauty-salon treatments
• faradic toning

- full-body massage
- galvanic treatment
- infra-red treatment
- manicure
- paraffin wax treatment
- Sixtus alpine plant footcare treatments
- Ultrabronze sunbeds
- universal contour wraps
- vacuum suction
- waxing (face, leg and underarm)

> **AVERAGE PRICE**
>
> Five-day Slimaway
> 🌷🌷🌷🌷🌷🌷🌷
>
> Seven-day Slimaway
> 🌷🌷🌷🌷🌷🌷🌷
> 🌷🌷🌷

## SPRINGS HYDRO

*Arlick Farm, Packington, nr. Ashby de la Zouch, Leicestershire*
*LE6 5TG*
*Telephone: (0530) 73873*

Part of the Henlow Grange group, Springs is set in rolling countryside close to an ancient spa town. Not only is it Britain's newest and first purpose-built health hydro, but everything about the resort has been designed specifically to create an atmosphere of restful, relaxing tranquillity. Smaller than the average hydro (with only 41 bedrooms), Springs nonetheless incorporates a number of extra touches of luxury that ensure its place as a worthy competitor to some of the more established resorts.

Among Springs' regular clientele are a number of sports personalities, television celebrities, executives and business people.

Free sporting, fitness and recreational facilities include:
- bicycles
- bowling green
- creative sculpture
- croquet
- evening lectures
- golf driving range
- gymnasium with the latest fitness and toning equipment
- indoor swimming pool complex with saunas, steamrooms,

plunge, whirl and splash pools
• jazz classes
• jogging sessions
• pitch and putt
• step workout
• tennis
• terrain bikes
• water exercises
• yoga, aerobics and relaxation classes

Available at extra charge are private swimming lessons; tennis, golf and archery coaching; personal training and fitness assessments; and physiotherapy. Horse-riding, golf and squash can be arranged locally, also at additional cost.

Inclusive in tariff:
Massage and facial on day of arrival, and one massage daily thereafter. However, there are a range of special promotional packages whose tariffs may include a greater number of inclusive daily treatments.

Optional extras:
• aroma and reflex-zone treatments
• aroma massage
• aromatherapy
• auto tan
• beauty-salon and hair treatments (including a range of special facials)
• BMR (basal metabolic rate) and fitness testing
• body wraps
• bust modelling
• cholesterol testing
• collagen treatments
• faradic treatments
• floatation room
• G5
• gommage (exfoliating body scrub) and massage

- hydrotherapy
- manicures
- Medichek
- nail extensions
- natural healing therapies
- pedicures
- remedial massage
- toning tables
- waxing

## STOBO CASTLE HEALTH SPA

*Stobo Castle, Peeblesshire, Scotland EH45 8NY*
*Telephone: (0721) 760249*

Set in the heart of the historic Borders, 27 miles south of Edinburgh and close to the famous river Tweed, Stobo Castle literally reeks of history. Although the present castle is only 200 years old, the Manor of Stobo itself dates back over 1,000 years, and the grace and nobility of the building make it difficult not to imagine that you are treading in the footsteps of former Scottish nobles and pretenders to the throne. Despite the imposing grandeur of the exquisitely panelled public rooms and sweeping staircase, Stobo has a reputation of being a warm and friendly resort that attracts swarms of wealthy people.

Free sporting, fitness and recreational facilities include:
- chef's demonstrations
- cycling
- evening entertainments
- exercise and dance classes
- guided walks
- gymnasium
- heated indoor pool
- nature trails
- tennis
- whirlpool

Golf, horse riding, and fly and coarse fishing can be arranged at extra cost.

Inclusive in tariff:

This varies according to the type of break booked. For example, on a two-night Holiday Plan break the price will include one heat treatment and body massage daily, whereas the Health and Beauty or Health and Fitness plans each incorporate five daily treatments in a two-day break, and between seven and ten daily treatments if seven days are booked.

Optional extras:
- acumassage
- algotherapy
- aromatherapy (with or without infra–red treatment)
- beauty-salon and hair treatments (including a range of special facials, collagen, bust and body treatments, electrolysis, skin analysis, manicure and pedicure)
- cool stocking treatment
- depilatory waxing
- Ionithermie
- massage (hand, underwater, remedial, vibratory etc.)
- Massaroma
- moor peat bath
- parafango and paraffin waxing
- reflexology
- sauna
- Slendertone
- spa baths
- sun beds
- Thalgo plasma gel and seaweed baths
- Ultratone
- Vacusager

TYRINGHAM NATUROPATHIC CLINIC
*Newport Pagnell, Buckinghamshire MK16 9ER*
*Telephone: (0908) 610450*
As a registered charity (and registered nursing home) operat-

---

**AVERAGE PRICE**

Per night – from
🌷🌷🌷🌷🌷

ing on a non-profit-making basis, Tyringham Naturopathic Clinic is in a slightly different league to most other British health resorts. Set in a secluded Georgian mansion amidst 30 acres of gardens, woodlands and surrounding farmland, the special nature of Tyringham's philosophy of treatment tends mainly to attract two types of people – those who are dedicated to naturopathic principles of health treatment, and those who are seeking treatment or cures for medical and health problems of a more chronic nature.

With the emphasis on treatment based on sound naturopathic principles, Tyringham accepts clients on a minimum stay of one week; but as it prefers to offer treatment on a longer-term basis, it recommends a stay of three or four weeks. A special Needy Patient's Fund offers generous reductions to patients who would otherwise not be able to afford treatment.

Free sporting, fitness and recreational facilities include:
- badminton
- crazy golf
- croquet
- film and fashion shows
- games room
- outdoor pool
- putting
- table tennis
- tennis

Inclusive in tariff:

All consultations and treatments as prescribed. Separate charges are made for X-rays, blood tests, ECGs and homoeopathic and herbal medicines.

Treatments include:
- acupuncture techniques (including laser, electro, moxibustion and TENS)
- heat and ice packs
- hydrotherapy (including Sitz baths, Scottish douche, salt water and mineral baths, whirlpool and sauna)

- massage (neuro-muscular, Swedish and vibro-massage)
- negative ionisation
- osteopathy
- physiotherapy and electrical muscle stimulation
- pressure drainage
- sauna, steam and radiant heat baths
- stress-release instruction
- tonic treatments (including respiration and breathing exercises, herbal oil and essence inhalation and remedial exercise)
- yoga

Optional extras:
Beauty, cosmetic and hair treatments.

**AVERAGE PRICE**

**Per week**

❀❀❀❀❀❀
❀❀❀

# THE UNITED STATES

In the United States, health havens are not called 'hydros' or 'fat farms', but by their traditional name: 'spas'. And because virtually everyone in the United States has embraced the whole concept of healthy living, American spas have been made deliberately accessible to all types of people with incomes ranging from the modest to the 'mega', by categorising themselves into four different kinds of experience: the 'resort', the 'fitness', the 'budget', and the 'one-day' spa.

## Resort Spas

According to America's most prominent health and fitness magazine, *Longevity*, 'resort' spas tend to be those that 'integrate the spa experience into a more traditional vacation'. Here, clients are allowed to pick and choose how much or how little advantage they take of traditional 'spa' life. They may opt for either the 'spa package' with a set number of treatments included in the price, or to pay a simple nightly room rate and take their pick of available treatments on an *à la carte* basis. Some resort spas offer family nutrition programmes, and special activities for

the kids. You can take unlimited advantage of all the extra free
activities provided as an integral feature of most vacational resorts
regardless of whether you avail yourselves of the sumptuous array
of treatments on offer.

Below are listed a few out of a vast selection of American
resort spas.

BONAVENTURA RESORT AND SPA
*Fort Lauderdale, Florida*
*Telephone: (305) 389 3300*
Average Price: One week $1,700–$2,500

FOUR SEASONS RESORT AND CLUB
*Las Colinas, Dallas, Texas*
*Telephone: (800) 332 3442*
Average Price: 6 nights – $1,500–$2,000

THE LODGE AT BRECKENRIDGE
*Breckenridge, Colorado*
*Telephone: (800) 736 1607*
Average Price: 1 week – $1,550

PGA NATIONAL RESORT AND SPA
*Palm Beach Gardens, Florida*
*Telephone: (800) 633 9150*
Average Price: 4 days – $875–$2,000

THE PHOENICIAN
*Scotsdale, Arizona*
*Telephone: (800) 888 8234*
Average Price: 1 week – $1,675–$2,500 (spa faciliies around
$500 extra)

SONOMA MISSION INN AND SPA
*Sonoma, California*
*Telephone: (707) 938 9000*
Average Price: 5 days – $1,000–$2,000

## Fitness Spas

Less pampering, more outdoor exercise (especially hiking) is the theme of many American 'fitness' spas. Some are classed as 'moveable spas' in that they consist of custom-designed hiking trips to spectacular locations such as the island of Maui (Hawaii), Arizona and Montana (known as 'Big Sky country' to Americans for its wide open spaces and incredible scenery that stretches as far as the eye can see).

THE ASHRAM
*Calabasas, California*
*Telephone: (818) 222 6900*
Average Price: 1 week – $2,000+ (including a few spa services)

CANYON RANCH HEALTH & FITNESS RESORT
*Tucson, Arizona*
*Telephone: (800) 742 9000*
Average Price: 1 week – $2,500+

THE CHALLENGES (MOVEABLE SPA)
*At Gurney's Inn and Spa Resort, New York (plus other locations)*
*Telephone: (800) 448 9816*
Average Price
1 week – $2,000+ (spa facilities extra)

GLOBAL FITNESS ADVENTURES (MOVEABLE SPA)
*Telephone: (800) 488 8747*
Average Price
1 week – $1,750–$2,000 (inclusive of some spa services)

NEW LIFE FITNESS VACATIONS
*Killington, Vermont*
*Telephone: (800) 228 4676*
Average Price: 1 week – $1,000–$1,250 (inclusive of some spa facilities)

THE PHOENIX SPA
*Houston, Texas*
*Telephone: (800) 548 4700*
Average Price: 6 nights – $1,500 +

RANCHO LA PEURTA
*Baja California, Mexico*
*Telephone: (800) 443 7565*
Average Price: 1 week – $1,275–$2,000 (spa facilities extra)

SAFETY HARBOR SPA & FITNESS CENTER
*Safety Harbor, Florida*
*Telephone: (800) 237 0155*
Average Price: 1 week – $1,500–$2,000

TOPNOTCH AT STOWE RESORT AND SPA
*Stowe, Vermont*
*Telephone: (800) 451 8686*
Average Price: 1 week – $1,300–$1,750 (including some
spa services)

## Budget Spas

As you might expect from their name, 'budget' spas are pretty
cheap. While they may not have the same range of equipment
as their more costly rivals, they still offer quite a variety of
treatments. The catch is that most of these are only available
on an à la carte basis, so if you think you may not be able to
resist the temptation to take advantage of one or two, you
should make allowances for any potential 'extras' in your
budget. If you are prepared to sacrifice your privacy you could
cut the overall basic price of your stay quite considerably by
sharing a 'dormitory-style' room.

All the prices quoted below should be taken as an approximate guide only. However, all are likely to include at least five
spa treatments, apart from those marked 'some spa facilities' in
which case you can expect to receive fewer treatments than five.

DEERFIELD MANOR SPA
*East Stroudsburg, Pennsylvania*
*Telephone: (800) 847 5637*
Average Price
1 week — $700–$1,000 (spa extra)

LAKE AUSTIN RESORT
*Austin, Texas*
*Telephone: (800) 847 5637*
Average Price: 1 week — $1,000–$1,250 (spa extra)

NATIONAL INSTITUTE OF FITNESS
*Ivins, Utah*
*Telephone: (801) 673 4905*
Average Price: 6 nights — $550–$1,100 (spa extra)

NEW AGE HEALTH SPA
*Neversink, New York*
*Telephone: (800) 682 4348*
Average Price: 1 week — $600–$1,250 (spa extra)

THE OAKS AT OJAI
*Ojai, California*
*Telephone: (805) 646 5573*
Average Price: 1 week — $875–$1,250 (including some spa
services)

THE PALMS AT PALM SPRINGS
*Palm Springs, California*
*Telephone: (619) 325 1111*
Average Price: 1 week — $1,050–$1,900

THE PLANTATION SPA
*Oahu, Hawaii*
*Telephone: (808) 237 8685*
Average Price: 6 nights — $1,150–$1,500 (including some
spa services)

RIO CALIENTE
*Guadalajara, Jalisco, Mexico*
*Telephone: (818) 796 5577*
Average Price: 1 week — $500–$1,000 (spa extra)

TENNESSEE FITNESS
*Waynesboro, Tennessee*
*Telephone: (800) 235 8365*
Average Price: 1 week — $500–$775 (spa extra)

## Day Spas

If you are in need of a little exercise or a quick revitalising session while on vacation in the United States or visiting from another state, you can visit one of the many 'day' spas that you will find in virtually every large city. You can book in for as little as one half-hour treatment, or you can take advantage of a treatment 'package': a half-day session should include three to four treatments; a full-day session should include five to six. Although the treatments are likely to cost a little more than you would expect to pay elsewhere, this type of break can be worth every penny for the weary traveller .

BEAUTY BODY WELLNESS
*San Francisco, California*
*Telephone: (415) 626 4685*
Average Price: Half day — $175+, full day — $290

BEAUTY KLINIEK
*San Diego, California*
*Telephone: (619) 457 0191*
Average Price: Half day — $100–$250, full day — $230–$350

BODIFERIER
*Greenwich, Connecticut*
*Telephone: (203) 698 1104*
Average Price: Half day — $95, full day - $150–$280

## THE CLAREMONT RESORT & SPA
*Oakland, California*
*Telephone: (510) 843 3000*
Average Price: Half day – $75, full day – $100–$285

## LE PLI AT THE HERITAGE
*Boston, Massachusetts*
*Telephone: (617) 426 6999*
Average Price: Half day – $175, full day – $315

## NORWICH INN & SPA
*Norwich, Connecticut*
*Telephone: (203) 886 2401*
Average Price: Full day – $200–$300

## THE OXFORD AVEDA SPA & SALON
*Denver, Colorado*
*Telephone: (303) 628 5435*
Average Price: Half day – $80–$100, full day – $185

## THE PENINSULA SPA
*New York, NY*
*Telephone: (212) – 903 3910*
Average Price: Full day – $175–$250

## PIERRE & CARLO EUROPEAN SPA SALON
*Philadelphia, PA*
*Telephone: (215) 790 9910*
Average Price: Half day – $175, full day – $250–$550

## URBAN RETREAT
*Houston, Texas*
*Telephone: (713) 523 2300*
Average Price: Full day – $95–$425

# EUROPEAN SPAS

The majority of European spas concentrate on health, beauty, fitness, recuperation following surgery or ill health, and the alleviation of pain. Certain spas specialise in treating specific problems or complaints, such as skin ailments, catarrh, bronchitis, back problems, heart disorders, dental problems, and smoking or alcohol addiction. Some European spas tend to attract their clientele from one or two specific countries, so unless you speak their language you might have trouble communicating with your fellow guests.

In addition, if you are visiting your chosen spa following illness or for specific medical or health reasons, it is always advisable to take along an explanatory letter from your doctor. Make sure that this is translated into the language of the country you are visiting, as many spa doctors tend to be local practitioners with little or no knowledge of English.

The following is just a small selection of European spas.

## *Austria*

GRAND HOTEL SAUERHOF (FIVE STAR)
*Baden, nr. Vienna*
A two-week spa package includes 10 massages, 10 special treatments, sulphur baths, and free use of indoor pool, sauna, solarium and tennis courts. One-week beauty packages are also available.

## *France*

GRAND HOTEL DES THERMES
*St. Malo*
Special thalassotherapy package available offering seven nights half-board plus three thalassotherapy treatments and use of all other facilities.

## DOMAINE DE REJAUBERT
*Dieulefit, Drôme-Provence*
Treatment focuses on relaxation and stress-relief, circulation problems and weight loss. Available treatments include an Ozotherm Ozone chamber, algotherapy, massage, hydro-massage, muscular hygiene, stretching, cosmetic care, Turkish bath, sauna, solaria and UVA tanning. Special seven-night 'Health and Beauty Treatment' packages include one health, facial and hair treatment daily for six days. 'Golf and Health' packages offer six days' worth of treatments for golfing enthusiasts, with green fees included in the price.

## HOTEL MIRAMAR (FIVE STAR)
*Biarritz*
Strongly recommended for the spa treatments it offers in conjunction with the Louison-Bobet Centre where all treatments are taken, this centre also appeals to golf enthusiasts wishing to combine their favourite sport with the healthy treatment options available at the centre.

## HOTEL THALAZUR
*Antibes*
The hotel has year-round access to the Institute of Thalassotherapy where the facilities include: covered seawater swimming pools heated by jet streams, two seawater pools for leisure and sports training, solarium, exercise rooms, algae baths, massage, aerosol therapy, acupuncture, tennis, gymnastics and beauty-therapy treatments.

The Institute specialises in fitness training, post-maternity recuperation, and providing treatments for cellulite, obesity, metabolic disturbances, gout, high cholesterol, rheumatic illnesses, stress, depression, early ageing, and deficiency illnesses.

# Germany

## HOTEL TOELZERHOF
*Bad Toelz*
Situated in the Bavarian Alps, this hotel offers special health-package stays from 7–28 days. These specialise in the treatment of arthritis, rheumatism, spinal problems, arterial disease, circulation disorders and patients convalescing from illness and/or surgery. Facilities include medical baths, massages, a range of beauty treatments and leisure options including golf, painting and tennis.

# Italy

## CASTLE RUNDEGG HEALTH FARM
*Merano*
A luxury establishment housed in an old converted castle. Treatments at the 'Fitness Palace' include mud packs, physiotherapy, underwater massage, lymphatic drainage, epidermic testing, inhalations, acupuncture, 'cures' for alcoholics, Finnish sauna and solarium. Castle Rundegg also houses a 'Beauty Palace' where clients can take advantage of virtually every beauty treatment ever invented.

## PALACE SPA HOTEL (FOUR STAR)
*Merano*
This hotel runs a selection of special 14-day Thermal Cures/Diet Programme packages. These include six mud pack treatments, 6 radon baths, 6 massages, a drink 'cure', half-hour gymnastic sessions, swimming, sauna, hot whirlpool bath, and Kneipp treatment.

## JOLLY HOTEL (FOUR STAR)
*Ischia*
This is just one of 70 spa establishments based on the beautiful island of Ischia, which is renowned both for its hot springs (whose fame goes back to Homer and Virgil), and also for the

fact that it is the oldest Greek Colony in the western Mediterranean, dating back 800 years BC. The Hotel Jolly offers an excellent thermal section with over 100 treatment booths, two thermal pools, a fresh-water pool for children, Finnish sauna, gymnasium, beauty parlour and cinema. Treatments include physiotherapy, kinesitherapy, massage, sauna and individually prescribed diets.

## Spain

HOTEL BYBLOS
*Mijas Golf, nr. Malaga*
On the sunny Costa del Sol, this hotel has a 'Louison-Bobet' spa section where thalassotherapy is available. Clients can take advantage of a special seven-night spa package which includes a number of treatments, or a seven-night golf package which includes green fees at two nearby 18-hole courses and a massage.

## Switzerland

Health spas abound in Switzerland, some of which even combine special spa and skiing packages.

BADEN, NR. ZURICH
Baden is said to be a delightful little town rich in thermal springs and minerals, with a special 'spa zone' area where a number of hotels are directly connected to the spa treatment centre. Both the four-star de luxe Hotel Staadhof and the four-star first-class Hotel Verenahof provide excellent bases for clients taking advantage of the special Baden packages. These include: The Baden Unwind Package, which offers a one week Anti-Stress programme; The Baden Health Programme, which combines a two- or three-week stay with 13–20 thermal baths, and 5–7 Fango (mud pack) treatments under medical supervision; The Baden Beauty Programme, which comprises a one-week stay with several beauty treatments run coopera-

tively with Lancome Beauty Products; and the Baden Anti-
Smoking Therapy Package, which condenses a broad-based
medical and scientific approach, applying techniques of
psychotherapy, behavour therapy and learning psychology into
a five- to eight-day treatment for those who have been smoking for 10 years or more.

LEUKERBAD
*Loeche-Les-Bains*
Here you can take advantage of a five-day health programme
of spa treatments to help you regain your ski fitness. Treatments
include hydrotherapy, physiotherapy, kinesitherapy, Fango
packs, beauty treatments, gymnastics and yoga. You can devote
your spare time to open-air curling, skating, cross-country
skiing and alpine ski touring.

---

Details of a comprehensive selection of specialist spas,
health farms and thalasotherapy centres established in virtually every European country as well as Hawaii, the Caribbean,
California, Florida, Arizona and many other American states
can be obtained by contacting specialist travel consultant:
Erna Low Consultants Ltd., 9 Reece Mews, London SW7
3HE, telephone: (071) 584 2841/7820.

---

PART THREE

# *Vitamins, Minerals and Nutritional Therapy*

'**B**eauty', we often hear, 'is only skin deep'. This phrase has become a cliché and is rarely interpreted as meaning precisely what it says, but it should be. It should be taken quite literally by anyone with pretensions to attaining any of the external qualities that constitute 'beauty' today. For in the words of the world-famous nutritionist, Earl Mindell, 'What you look like on the outside depends a lot on what you do for yourself on the inside.' In other words, if you do not ensure that your internal body is provided with adequate nutrition then no amount of expensive treatments can ever help you succeed in your quest.

## NUTRITION AND HEALTH

Optimum nutrition is vital. Not only because it provides the body with all it needs to create and maintain strong bones, healthy tissues, a good musculature, glossy hair and youthful-looking skin, but also because it effectively provides the body with *everything* it needs in order to function.

All of us would like to live forever, or at least to enjoy a ripe, healthy old age. And if we can retain our looks and our mental faculties, too, then so much the better. According to world-famous naturopath and osteopath, Leon Chaitow, every human being is born with the potential not only to exceed his or her prescribed 'four score years and ten' by a very long chalk, but also to retain the health and vitality to enjoy each and every one of them.

The accepted scientific formula for calculating how long all mammal species live (and humans are mammals, too) is to multiply by five the time it takes the skeleton to mature. In humans, skeletal development is complete by the age of 25. Multiplying this figure by five, therefore, gives us a potential lifespan of 125 years. Left to their own devices, our genes might allow many of us to do just that. Unfortunately, there are many factors that have a combined negative effect on our looks, our health and our potential lifespan, including chemical pollution, stress, toxins, infections and, especially, nutritional deficiency.

While we may not be able to do much on our own to alter many of the external environmental influences, we can and should ensure that we retain full control over our nutritional intake. Good nutrition can do much both to mitigate the effects of negative lifestyle influences and to significantly improve our prospects for a longer, healthier and more beautiful life.

## Free Radicals

Scientists have recently identified certain major factors in the ageing process and the development of disease. One of the most significant is the harmful biochemical process caused by 'free radicals'. These extremely aggressive chemical compounds harm the body by invading its cells and destroying their thin, outer membranes that protect them against attack from toxic substances and disease. Once inside, free radicals commence to destroy the DNA in the cell nucleus and so spark off the process that leads to a general lowering of our defences against ageing and disease. In fact, free radicals have now been identified as major contributory factors to the development of more than 200 well-known serious diseases.

Pollution, smoking, excessive amounts of fats in the diet, high blood pressure and stress can all contribute to the formation of excessive numbers of free radicals in the body. Although the body's in-built defence mechanism can create certain enzymes to protect itself against free radicals, this can work efficiently only if the diet contains sufficient amounts of 'antioxidant' vitamins and minerals. These include vitamins C and E, beta carotene, selenium and other trace elements such as zinc, manganese and copper.

# VITAMINS

Vitamins are essential for normal growth and maintenance of

the body tissues. They are also responsible for the normal metabolism of other nutrients. As the body cannot synthesise most vitamins, these must be obtained from food. In general, only very small amounts are needed as their functions are primarily catalytic, as components of enzyme systems involved in metabolic reactions.

Although most foods contain a variety of vitamins, no single food contains *all* the vitamins required. This is why a diet derived from a wide range of foods is recommended. Individual vitamins vary greatly both in chemical composition and in their functions.

## Vitamin A (Retinol)

Vitamin A is fat-soluble, which means that it requires fats as well as minerals for proper absorption by the digestive tract. The fact that it can also be stored by the body means that it need not be ingested every day. This vitamin is essential for several vital functions.

Children need vitamin A in order to grow, as it plays an important role in many of the body processes necessary for healthy growth to occur. Vitamin A is also essential for normal vision, and is particularly important to the light-receptor cells called rods and cones in the retina of the eye. The first sign of a deficiency is poor night vision, which is why carrots (which are an excellent source of this vitamin) are said to help you 'see in the dark'. The acute form of this condition, known as xerophthalmia, is a widespread problem in the developing world and, unless corrected by administration of Vitamin A, can lead to permanent loss of vision.

Other functions for which Vitamin A is essential are reproduction, and maintenance of the structure and health of bones, skin, teeth, gums and mucous membranes.

In the liver of a well-nourished adult, vitamin A stores can supply the body's needs for many months. It is unlikely that anyone on a normal diet could 'overdose' on this vitamin, but care should be taken when using supplements. Large amounts of vitamin A can exceed the liver's capacity to store the vitamin, resulting in adverse effects on the body.

In Britain, the recommended daily intake of vitamin A is 700 micrograms (mcg) for men and 600 mcg for women, with a lower level for children. Women who are pregnant or breastfeeding are advised to increase their intake. Liver is a a very rich source of Retinol and those who never eat it will depend more heavily on vegetables, which may contribute as much as 50 per cent of their vitamin-A requirements.

Half of the daily Reference Nutrient Intake (RNI for males 19–50 years) can be found in any of the following:
- 7 ounces (200 grams) of cantaloupe melon
- 3 ounces (85 grams) of watercress
- 2 ounces (57 grams) of dried apricots
- 4 ounces (113 grams) of Cheddar cheese

A full day's amount can be obtained from 3 ounces (85 grams) of spinach, or just 2 ounces (57 grams) of carrots.

Best sources:
- margarine fortified with vitamin A
- liver
- oily fish
- dairy products

Although deficiency in vitamin A is rare in the West, there are a number of factors that may adversely affect levels of the vitamin in the body:

1) Dietary factors such as a low fat intake will adversely affect the metabolism and absorption of carotenoids.
2) Acute infections appear to lower concentrations of vitamin A in the blood and may also deplete liver reserves.

Symptoms of deficiency include:
- dry skin
- night blindness
- xeropthalmia

## Beta Carotene

Exciting new research and many epidemiological studies show that carotenoids and, in particular, beta carotene, act as protective agents in the diet and may prevent or delay the development of cancerous tumours. Carefully controlled trials are underway and results should be known within the next few years. In the light of these developments, the USA National Research Council is already recommending that consumption of fruits and carotene-rich vegetables is increased.

Beta carotene is a precursor of vitamin A which can be converted into the active vitamin in the body. Unlike vitamin A, however, it is not possible to overdose on beta carotene because it is converted in the body only at the rate at which it is needed. The best sources are all orange, yellow, red and green fruits and vegetables, especially carrots.

## Vitamin B1*(Thiamin)

Vitamin B1 is essential for growth, healthy muscles and the nervous system. It is also required for the conversion of carbohydrates into energy, which is why those on high-carbohy- drate diets require high intakes of the vitamin. Like all the B-complex vitamins, any excess of thiamin is not stored in the body, but excreted, and for this reason should be replenished daily.

Best sources:
- milk
- meat
- soya beans
- poultry
- wholegrain and fortified cereals
- peanuts
- pork
- green vegetables
- yeast

*All the B Vitamins work synergistically. That is to say, they are more potent when taken together than when used separately. To work effectively, Earl Mindell recommends that B1, B2 and B6 be equally balanced.

Studies have shown that teenagers and the elderly tend to have lower intakes of thiamin than other groups because they eat too many starchy foods and snacks. Our daily need depends on the amount of carbohydrate we eat and how active we are. The Reference Nutrient Intake (RNI) for adult males is 0.1 milligrams. However, pregnant women, the elderly, heavy drinkers or those with a sweet tooth (who may take most of their carbohydrate as sugars) may need more. Thiamin is easily lost during preparation and cooking of foods – grilling, for example, can cause a loss of up to 40 per cent of the nutrient.

Historically, thiamin deficiency occurred in people subsisting on diets of mainly white rice, and the deficiency disease 'beriberi' was responsible for the death of hundreds of thousands of people earlier this century.

Symptoms of deficiency include:
- beriberi
- muscle weakness
- Wernicke's encephalopathy

## Vitamin B2 (Riboflavin)

This vitamin plays an essential role in all oxidative processes in the body, and aids in growth and reproduction. It is necessary for healthy skin, nails, hair, mouth, eyes and general wellbeing, and is particularly important during pregnancy or when breast-feeding. As it is not stored in the body, we need regular dietary supplies. The RNI for Riboflavin for teenagers and females over 18 is 1.3 mg; for adult males.

Best sources:
- milk
- meat
- fortified cereals
- wheatgerm
- soya beans
- eggs
- green vegetables

As milk is a major source of this vitamin, deficiencies are widespread in countries where dairy products are not regularly consumed. Riboflavin is light sensitive – half of it can, for example, disappear from milk after a couple of hours in bright sunlight.

Symptoms of deficiency include:

- chapped lips
- sore tongue
- skin rashes
- non-specific symptoms such as fatigue and inability to work

Severe deficiency may result in glossitis, dermatitis and cheilosis.

## *Vitamin B3\*(Niacin)*

This vitamin plays a critical role in numerous biochemical processes, notably energy metabolism. It is also essential for growth, digestion of carbohydrates, and healthy skin and nervous system. Niacin can be synthesised in the body from tryptophan, one of the amino acids in protein. The RNI is 17 mg but women may need extra supplies during later months of pregnancy and whilst breast-feeding.

Best sources:

- fish
- liver
- meat
- poultry
- wholegrains
- peanuts
- breakfast cereals
- eggs

*In Britain and the United States, niacin (nicotinic acid, nicotinamide or niacinamide) is known as Vitamin B3, whilst in some European countries this number is accorded to pantothenic acid, which is known as B5 to the British and Americans. In order to avoid confusion, niacin and pantothenic acid should be referred to by their names, and not their numbers.

Deficiency of this vitamin was responsible for the disease pellagra which was widespread in southern parts of the United States and Europe up to 50 years ago. Symptoms are diarrhoea, skin diseases and dementia. Although niacin is relatively stable, losses can occur when food is blanched.

Symptoms of deficiency:
- pellagra
- dermatitis
- diarrhoea
- mental disturbance
- mucosal lesions
- anorexia

## Vitamin B5 (Pantothenic Acid, Calcium Pantothenate)

Pantothenic acid is essential for healthy growth, the building of cells, development of the central nervous system, proper functioning of the adrenal glands, synthesis of hormones and production of antibodies. It is also involved in the metabolism of food.

Best sources:
- liver
- eggs
- wholemeal bread
- brown rice
- yeast-based products

Present in almost every type of food, pantothenic acid is fairly stable during ordinary cooking and storage. Some methods of processing foods, however, such as those involving high temperatures or acidic or alkaline conditions, can cause considerable losses. Intakes of pantothenic acid vary widely but on average are somewhere between 4–6 mg daily. There is no currently established RNI in Britain and no evidence of gross deficiencies, although it has been suggested that the diet may be inadequate in certain groups such as pregnant teenagers.

Symptoms of deficiency:
• hypoglycaemia
• duodenal ulcers
• blood and skin disorders

## *Vitamin B6 (Pyridoxine)*

This vitamin is involved at almost every stage in protein metabolism (hence requirements are related to protein intake). Pyridoxine also helps the body to metabolise certain fats, and is essential for the metabolism of protein, and for the health of skin, muscles and the entire nervous system.

Best sources:
• fish
• poultry
• meat
• eggs
• peanuts
• cereals
• green vegetables
• yeast
• wheatgerm

For most adults, a daily intake of 1.4 mg is sufficient, although this should be increased during pregnancy and while breast-feeding. It is commonly taken as a supplement by women concerned about premenstrual tension (PMT).

Symptoms of deficiency:
• macrocytic anaemia
• dermatitis
• depression
• peripheral neuritis

## Vitamin B12 (Cyanocobalamin)

Essential in the metabolism of folate and of amino, fatty and nucleic acids (DNA and RNA), vitamin B12 also aids the formation of red blood cells, and contributes to growth and a healthy nervous system. This B-vitamin is unusual in that tissue reserves last for as long as three to five years. Only very small amounts are required on a daily basis and all foods derived from animals are good sources.

Best sources:
- meat, especially organ meats such as liver and kidneys
- fish
- eggs
- dairy products

The metabolic functions of B12 are closely associated with those of folic acid, and a deficiency causes the same type of anaemia. The only people at risk of deficiency, however, are vegans (strict vegetarians who eat no animal products, including dairy foods). For vegans, a regular supplement is recommended. Supplements may also be necessary when absorption is impaired, which can occur in the elderly.

Symptoms of deficiency:
- macrocytic anaemia
- peripheral neuritis

## Folic Acid (Folate)

Also part of the B-complex group of vitamins, folic acid is required for the metabolism of some amino acids and for the synthesis of nucleic acids. It helps in the formation of new body cells, particularly red blood cells. Only very small amounts of folic acid are required daily, but bear in mind that the vitamin is destroyed by cooking and prolonged storage.

Best sources:
- liver and other offal meats
- leafy green vegetables

- fortified cereals
- yeast

Deficiencies of this vitamin do occur in Britain and other countries, and cause a form of anaemia in young children, the elderly and pregnant women, as well as gastrointestinal disorders. Supplements are frequently prescribed in pregnancy, especially since new evidence has arisen linking deficiency in folic acid with the potential development of neural-tube defects such as spina bifida.

Symptoms of deficiency:
- anaemia
- macrocytic anaemia

## Biotin

The eighth member of the B-complex group of vitamins, biotin is involved in the metabolism of carbohydrates and fats. According to Earl Mindell, biotin helps prevent baldness and grey hair, eases muscle pain and alleviates eczema and dermatitis. No RNI for biotin has yet been established.

Best sources
- nuts
- fruits
- brewer's yeast
- beef liver
- egg yolk
- milk
- kidney
- unrefined rice

There is no evidence of biotin deficiency in humans on normal, mixed diets. In experimental deficiencies in humans, skin lesions were the first signs to appear. Earl Mindell states that Biotin deficiency can cause extreme exhaustion and impair fat metabolism.

## Vitamin C (Ascorbic Acid)

Required for the formation of neurotransmitters and of collagen, vitamin C also increases absorption of iron from non-meat
sources and functions as an antioxidant. It is also essential for
the growth and repair of body-tissue cells, blood vessels, gums,
bones and teeth.

Best sources:
- citrus fruits
- cabbage
- potatoes
- salad vegetables
- tomatoes
- berries

Vitamin C is used up more rapidly under conditions of stress,
while tobacco is estimated to destroy Vitamin C at the rate
of 25 mg per cigarette smoked.

Symptoms of deficiency:
- scurvy
- sore gums
- capillary bleeding

## Vitamin D (Cholecalciferol)

Vitamin D is unlike other vitamins in that our bodies have the
ability to manufacture sufficient amounts to meet our daily
needs. Vitamin D is produced when sunlight converts a
substance present in our skin into cholecalciferol (a form of
vitamin D). No dietary sources are said to be necessary for
children and adults who are sufficiently exposed to sunlight,
but as this commodity is often lacking during the winter
months, it is especially important to pay particular attention
to our diet during this season and possibly take supplements.

As well as being important for our general wellbeing, vitamin D is, along with calcium, essential for strong, healthy
bones and teeth. It is therefore important that babies and grow-

ing children have adequate supplies. Mothers-to-be also need this vitamin to ensure that unborn babies' bones develop properly, whilst nursing mothers are often advised to increase their intake from food.

Only a few foods contain vitamin D, but small amounts of such foods are enough to supply a daily intake sufficient for good health. Just one ounce (28 grams) of margarine (to which vitamin D is added during manufacture) is sufficient, as is the same amount of kipper, herring or canned salmon, or two eggs.

Best sources:
• fortified margarine
• eggs
• fish-liver oils
• oily fish such as salmon, sardines, herring, tuna and mackerel
• dairy products

There is evidence to suggest that levels of vitamin D are lower in many old people, particularly in those over the age of 65 and those who are housebound. Evidence also suggests that a diet rich in vitamin D may help to strengthen brittle bones brought on by the menopause and old age.

Symptoms of deficiency:
• rickets
• bone deformities
• tetany
• severe tooth decay
• osteomalacia
• senile osteoporosis

## Vitamin E (Tocopherol)

The function of vitamin E has been of great interest and study ever since its discovery in 1922. It is now known that this vitamin is one of the most efficient natural antioxidants, and is found in tissue membranes both within and around every living cell. Currently the major research interest in this vitamin is its function in protecting against disease.

Requirements for this vitamin are related to dietary intake of polyunsaturated fats. The higher your intake, the more vitamin E you may need to prevent rancidification of the oils. Vitamin E is stored in the liver, fatty tissues, heart, muscles, testes, uterus, blood, adrenal and pituitary glands, but unlike other fat-soluble vitamins, it can be stored for only a relatively short time.

Vitamin E enhances the activity of vitamin A, and is claimed by many anti-ageing experts to help retard cellular ageing due to oxidation, and to play an important preventive role in coronary heart disease. It also appears to be of value in some premature infants to prevent brain haemorrhage, and recent research has suggested that it may have some benefits in the treatment of patients with early Parkinson's disease. Although the British Department of Health has not set a Recommended Daily Amount, current evidence suggests that a daily intake of about 5–10 mg is desirable.

Best sources:
- vegetable oils
- margarine
- green vegetables
- wheat germ
- soya beans
- whole-wheat
- whole-grain cereals
- eggs

As the concentration of vitamin E is higher in the blood of non-smokers than smokers, our requirements may be increased by smoking and by environmental pollution.

Symptoms of deficiency:
- neuromuscular dysfunction
- reduced lifespan of red blood cells
- some anaemias
- reproductive disorders

## Vitamin K (Phylloquinone)

This vitamin is essential for synthesis of prothrombin and maintenance of normal blood-clotting mechanisms.

Best sources:
- green salad vegetables
- vegetables
- potatoes
- tomatoes
- liver and liver oils
- soyabean oil
- kelp
- alfalfa
- egg yolk
- yoghurt

Symptoms of deficiency:
- abnormal blood clotting
- a fall in prothrombin content of the blood

According to Earl Mindell (who also refers to this vitamin as menadione), deficiency may also be a contributory factor to coeliac disease, sprue and colitis.

# MINERALS

Certain mineral elements are essential for life. Of these, calcium and phosphorus are the most important.

## Calcium

Needed for the formation and maintenance of healthy bones and teeth, calcium also plays a vital role in blood clotting and cellular signal transmission. People on a high-protein diet need a higher intake of calcium.

Best sources:
• dairy products
• fortified bread
• hard water
• dark-green leafy vegetables

In conjunction with a deficiency of vitamin D, too little calcium in the body may lead to rickets in children and osteomalacia in adults. Calcium deficiency may also contribute to the development of osteoporosis, and extreme deficiency (hypocalaemia) causes tetany.

## Magnesium

Required for skeletal development and the maintenance of electrical potential in nerve and muscle membranes, magnesium is also important for converting blood sugar into energy.
Best sources:
• green vegetables
• cereals
• meat
• nuts
• figs
• yellow corn
• seeds

Symptoms of deficiency:
• muscle weakness
• failure to thrive
• tachycardia
• anorexia
• neuromuscular changes

## Phosphorus

Present in every body cell, phosphorous is an important component of skeletal tissue. Phosphate compounds are required for the transfer of energy in muscle tissue, and are involved in virtually all physiological chemical reactions within the body. The mineral also plays an important role in regulating the heart, and is necessary for the formation and maintenance of normal bone and tooth structure; for the assimilation of niacin (vitamin B3); and for normal kidney function.

Although present in nearly all foods, best sources of phosphorus include:

- fish
- poultry
- meat
- whole grains
- eggs
- nuts
- seeds
- cereals
- protein-rich foods

Although phosphorus deficiency is pretty rare, symptoms include:

- feeling easily fatigued
- weakness
- decreased attention span

## Iron

Iron is essential for life and for the production of haemoglobin in the red-blood corpuscles which carry oxygen to the tissues. It also affects work capacity and immune function. Deficiency can lead to normocytic or microcytic hypochromic anaemia.

Best sources:

- offal
- egg yolks
- oysters
- nuts
- molasses
- beans
- oatmeal

- meat
- fish
- poultry
- fortified cereals

## Zinc

Present in all tissues and an essential component of many enzyme systems, zinc acts as a kind of traffic policeman in that it directs and oversees the efficient flow of body processes. It participates in the metabolism of nucleic acid and in the formation of insulin, and is essential for protein synthesis and the development and maintenance of the reproductive organs. Zinc is now also thought to be an important anti-oxidant nutrient.

Best sources:
- meat
- fish
- whole-grain cereals
- eggs
- wheat germ
- brewer's yeast
- pumpkin seeds
- skimmed dairy milk

Symptoms of deficiency:
- retarded growth
- immune dysfunction
- impaired healing

## Copper

Copper is required to convert the body's iron into haemoglobin, and it converts the amino acid tyrosine into the pigmenting factor for hair and skin. The mineral is also essential for the utilisation of vitamin C.

Best sources:
• dried beans
• peas
• whole-wheat
• prunes
• shrimps
• most seafood
• liver
• fish
• nuts

Symptoms of deficiency:
• leucopenia
• increased susceptibility to infections

## *Selenium*

This mineral is an important component of an antioxidant enzyme system which may protect intracellular structures. Selenium acts synergistically with vitamin E, another powerful free-radical scavenger. According to Earl Mindell, and other experts on nutrition, selenium may aid in: maintaining youthful elasticity in tissues; alleviating hot flushes and menopausal distress; treating and preventing dandruff; and possibly in neutralising certain carcinogens, thus providing protection against some forms of cancer.

Best sources:
• wheat germ
• bran
• tuna fish
• onions
• tomatoes
• broccoli
• cereals from hard wheat
• meat
• fish

## Chromium

Required for normal glucose metabolism, chromium also appears to potentiate the action of insulin, to bring protein to where it is needed, to aid growth, to help prevent and lower high blood pressure, and to work as a deterrent for diabetes. Chromium deficiency is a suspected factor in arteriosclerosis and diabetes.

Best sources:
- meat
- shellfish
- chicken
- corn oil
- clams
- brewer's yeast
- wholegrains
- nuts

## Iodine

This mineral forms part of the thyroid hormones which are necessary for the maintenance of metabolic rate and cellular metabolism.

Best sources:
- seafood
- fortified salt
- milk
- kelp
- vegetables grown in iodine-rich soil
- onions

Symptoms of deficiency:
- goitre
- hypothyroidism
- cretinism in children

## *Fluoride*

May have a role in bone mineralisation and protects against dental caries. Deficiency leads to tooth decay.
  Best sources:
  • fluoridated water
  • tea
  • seafoods
  • gelatin

# NUTRITIONAL THERAPY

Until recently, the idea of using vitamins and minerals to help treat or cure a number of physical and mental disorders was considered outlandish by all but a few dedicated researchers. Today, as more and more research is revealing the extent to which our bodies depend on optimum nutrition for effective functioning, even some of the most sceptical practitioners are beginning to regret their earlier dismissive attitude and to revise their opinion.

Experiments have shown, for example, that symptoms of mental illness can be switched on and off by altering vitamin levels in the body. The eminent Dr Linus Pauling, who was awarded a Nobel prize for his research into vitamin C (and is reported to take 13,000 mg himself every day), has not only conducted several series of tests to determine individual vitamin needs, but has also discovered that the mentally ill need a much greater amount of vitamin C than the rest of us.

In his widely respected and bestselling book, *The Vitamin Bible*, Earl Mindell reports that 'the following vitamins and minerals have, in many cases, been found to be effective in the treatment of depression and anxiety':
  • Vitamin B1 (thiamine) – large amounts appear to energise depressed people and tranquillise anxious ones
  • Vitamin B6 (pyridoxine) – important for the function of the adrenal cortex

- Pantothenic acid – has a tension-relieving effect
- Vitamin C (ascorbic acid) – essential for combating stress
- Vitamin E (alpha-tocopherol) – aids brain cells in getting their needed oxygen
- Zinc – oversees body processes and aids in brain function
- Magnesium – necessary for nerve functioning, known as the anti-stress mineral
- Calcium – makes you less jumpy, more relaxed.'

Furthermore, a whole range of naturally-derived substances are finally being subjected to scientific scrutiny. Double-blind trials are taking place in order to ascertain whether they do indeed have any inherent healing or curative powers, as centuries of herbalists and healers have always claimed, and, if they do, to investigate further precisely how and why they should. Substances being studied in this way include those derived from foods (such as garlic and onions), roots (ginseng and ginger), flowers (bee pollen and the evening primrose), leaves (ginkgo biloba extract), algae (spirulina and chlorella), sprouting beans (alfalfa leaves and seeds) and wheat and barley grass.

## Precautions

It seems that the secret of maintaining our youthful looks, vitality and energy throughout a long, extended, and supremely healthy life may reside totally in optimum nutrition, backed up by vitamin and mineral supplement therapy where required. Even if no one is quite ready to state this categorically, few experts in the scientific and medical fields are now refuting the possibility that this may indeed one day prove to be the case.

Until this supposition becomes fact, backed up by evidence and strict guidelines, it is still necessary to be guided by what is known, as opposed to what is claimed. For as we all know, our yearning for eternal youth, beauty and health can represent the biggest cloud of susceptibility that obscures our sense of balance, proportion, and logic about what is currently humanly possible, and what is not.

While vitamin and mineral therapy may appeal to many of us as a wholly natural approach to achieving our aim of prolonging our looks, our health, and our lives, it is important never to forget that even 'natural' therapies have their dangers. For this reason, I would strongly advise anyone interested in learning more about nutritional supplements firstly to become acquainted with all the facts that are currently available (see Recommended Reading, page 227); and secondly to obtain correct information regarding usage and safety in order to make informed choices about what should or should not be taken.

PART FOUR

# Anti-ageing Lotions, Potions Peels and Creams

T he mythical 'fountain of youth' has proved elusive. After centuries of fruitless quest, the cosmetics industry has tried to produce the next-best thing – a magical substance that might, if not quite prolong life indefinitely, at least provide a purely cosmetic approximation of the famed elixir to help us prolong our looks.

The first cosmetics empires were founded soon after the end of the First World War by Elizabeth Arden and Helena Rubinstein. Literally millions of women the world over have happily and hopefully contributed their own meagre portion to the several accumulated billions that have been spent on a series of ever-changing, new and improved, anti-ageing lotions, potions, peels and creams.

Every year, the giants of the cosmetics industry plough enough money into research and development to wipe out the national debts of several countries. Hundreds of chemists, cosmetologists and cosmetic scientists spend their days incarcerated in high-tech laboratories conducting experiments with a wide variety of natural and synthetic ingredients in the hope of finding the key that will unlock the secret of turning back time. Make no mistake – behind the scenes of every cosmetics empire a battle is being fought in a war as old as time itself for a prize as elusive as the Holy Grail.

Every few years, a new breakthrough is made, and try as they may to protect their latest discovery, no single cosmetics manufacturer has yet found it possible to keep its technology a secret. As soon as one company launches a brand-new anti-ageing formula, every one of its rivals hits back with their own 'unique' version. There can be few women today who have not tried anti-ageing facial creams based on liposomes, ceramide time capsules and nonionic lipid microspheres that promise to reduce lines and wrinkles by delivering their active ingredients right through to the living cells beneath the skin. We have bought age-defence systems containing collagen, elastin, fibrin, mucopolysaccharides, ginseng and free-radical scavenging vitamins such as C and E. We have tried youth serums based on Retin-A, and a whole series of acids with strange-sounding names such alpha-hydroxy, glycolic, hyaluronic and salicylic. And while few of us have a clue as to what any of these ingredients actually are, or even whether they really can create a permanent improvement in the appearance of our skin, we dip eagerly and ever-deeper into our pockets to find the not insignificant sums involved because, well, you never know... all that research must account for something.

The more advanced the technology behind facial rejuvenation creams becomes, the more confusing it is for us, the consumers, to understand precisely what each new wonder ingredient or innovation actually means. In order to protect their latest discoveries (and their profits), most manufacturers do not offer the consumer a precise breakdown of their products' ingredients, or even an adequate explanation of how or why it purports to work. Instead, they surround each new innovation with a tantalising mystique, using a vocabulary of long and unpronounceable pseudo-scientific words to endow it with credibility.

## LATEST PRODUCTS AND INGREDIENTS

In order to demystify some of the current jargon, here is a list of the latest 'buzz-words', together with what I hope is a simplified explanation of what each product or ingredient is, as well as the potential positive and negative effects it may have on the skin.

### *Alpha-hydroxy Acids*

Otherwise known as AHAs or 'fruit acids', these are a range, or 'family', of naturally occurring compounds discovered in the 1970s by American dermatologist Dr Eugene Van Scott. These substances include glycolic acid, which is found in sugar cane; lactic acid, which is made from fermented milk; citric and ascorbic acid (vitamin C), which come from citrus fruits and rose hips; pyruvic acid, which comes from papaya; malic acid, which comes from apples; and tartaric acid, which is made from grape wine.

The fact that Cleopatra was alleged to bathe in asses' milk to keep her skin young, soft and smooth indicates that the properties of 'fruit acids' have been known for a very long time. Indeed, records show that a number of primitive peoples have long made use of the peculiarly strong action caused by certain enzymes in fruits such as papaya by using the pulp of the fruit to tenderise meat.

When applied in low concentrations to the skin, fruit acids have a similar action to a chemical facial peel. Used regularly, they are claimed to have a super-effective exfoliating effect in that they gently strip away dead skin cells, revascularise tissue, promote new collagen formation, increase the production of healthy new skin cells, plump up the dermis and eliminate ageing lines and wrinkles.

Since their discovery by Van Scott, AHAs have been incorporated into dermatologist-prescribed creams with no known harmful side-effects. Dr Danné Montague-King, a doctor of pharmacology and leading botanical scientist, has been researching the benefits and uses of natural organic plant and herb extracts for skin regeneration for many years. He believes that AHAs work by swelling up the dead and dying cells of the skin like little balloons which then burst into fragments and detach from the skin. By dissolving the alkaline bonds that form a waxy substance that holds dead cells together (the intercellular glue), this action also promotes rapid exfoliation.

In the March 1992 edition of the British magazine, *Health and Beauty Salon*, Dr Montague-King writes:

> ... *the cells of the skin respond in a positive manner to chemistry the skin recognises, indeed chemistry it manufactures naturally on its own. Based on this principle, we find amino acids, other proteins, enzymes and fractioned oils from the plant world create an environment that allows living cells to remain alive a little bit longer, thus retarding the signs of ageing.*

*One of the first steps in skin care is to rid the epidermis of the dead cells build-up, often misconstrued as dry skin by cosmetic manufacturers. This barrier, medically categorised as redundant cuticle, not only appears as sallow, wrinkled, ageing skin on the surface, but actually slows down the normal activity of underlying new cell processes. These include the functions of the oil and sweat glands that provide us with that vital, moist acid mantle observed in young healthy skin.*

There are two methods of applying AHAs to the skin. The first is available in many forms of DIY facial cream preparations. Virtually every cosmetic manufacturer currently has its own preparation on the market, but many dermatologists are sceptical about their effectiveness, speculating that the dilute form used in some creams may render them inactive.

Meanwhile, however, all the big names in the cosmetic industry are launching their new AHA-based creams on a wave of remarkable claims. Not surprisingly, the majority of these are also being marketed at a remarkably inflated price. Here is a guide to what is currently available (tester's reports vary from the mildly encouraging to the downright disappointing):

• **Age Management Serum, by La Prairie**
  (from ♨ ♨ ♨ ♨ for 30 ml)

• **All You Need Action Moisturiser, by Prescriptives**
  (♨ ♨ ♨ for 50 ml)

• **Fruition Triple ReActivating Complex, by Estée Lauder**
  (from ♨ ♨ for 30 ml)

• **Ceramide Time Complex Moisture Cream, by Elizabeth Arden**
  (♨ ♨ ♨ for 50 ml)

• **Solution, by Avon**
  (♨ for 50 ml)

The second method of applying AHAs involves a professional facial peeling treatment. According to Dr Montague-King's promotional literature, 'the deep peel, suitable for very out of condition lined skin or acne scars, is the most effective treatment ever to be offered by beauty salons. A client with acne and scarred skin can expect to see an enormous reduction of scar tissue, pitting and spots. A smoother, fresher complexion will result with rejuvenated texture and colour.'

Ten days prior to treatment, a product called Retosin is used to prepare the skin. The actual procedure, which takes between one-and-a-half and two hours, involves the application of numerous layers of an AHA solution comprising glycolic, malic and citric acid to produce 'a controlled change in the skin', resulting in some redness and irritation. Within 24 hours of a 'peeling' treatment, the skin will begin to shed. Further appointments are required on the fifth and tenth days after treatment, the first to remove dead skin cells, and the second to undergo a further treatment session designed to leave the skin smooth and firm. Three weeks after the initial session, new collagen is said to be laid down which will mature in two months.

## *Results*

Descriptions of the sensations experienced during treatment range from 'strongly stinging' to 'painful but bearable'. But many testers report that their skin looks undeniably better after treatment than it did before.

Double-blind trials have been conducted by Dr Montague-King's top educator and research technician in Johannesburg, Ms Tracey Nathan. These involved direct delivery of his own AHA peeling serum to 50 clients, and revealed that the underlying collagen fibres in ageing skin became stronger after the initial treatment of fruit-sugar serum. Ms Nathan's carefully recorded notes and photographs also enabled her to deduce that, when the treatment was followed by heavy after-care with vitamin C, the skin's elasticity bounced back tighter and firmer.

## Collagen, Elastin & Hyaluronic Acid

**AVERAGE PRICE**

**Ranges from ♨♨♨ to ♨♨♨♨ for each facial (and you may require as many as four to achieve the desired effect) all the way up to ♨♨♨♨♨♨♨♨ ♨♨♨♨ for a fuller, deeper facial peel recommended for skin that is very wrinkled, or covered in acne scars. Either way, however, you can anticipate some drastic reddening and scabbing to take place.**

Young skin is remarkably elastic. When it is stretched it immediately springs back into place. As we age the skin begins to lose its springy flexibility with the result that wrinkles begin to appear. This effect is due to certain changes that take place in the collagen and elastin fibres of the connective tissue, and also to the progressive dehydration that occurs in mature skin.

Hyaluronic acid is a natural moisturising factor present in the dermis which helps bind water into the skin, and similarly protect it against water loss. As the amount of hyaluronic acid in the dermis declines with age, the skin becomes less efficient, not only at keeping water locked in, but also at preventing water loss.

Collagen synthesis begins in fibroblast cells when procollagen molecules are formed, each of which is made up of three chains of amino acids (known as polypeptide chains) that are coiled around each other. This triple helix structure is held together by hydrogen bonds which give the procollagen its considerable strength. When these molecules of procollagen leave the fibroblast cells they pass into the matrix of the connective tissue in the dermal layer where they arrange themselves lengthways in groups of five, held together by cross-links, to form microfibrils which, in turn, are combined into larger groups of fibrils.

Short chain lengths of collagen, prepared and derived from animal sources, are now being added to rejuvenating creams along with mucopolysaccharides which help to draw the lengths into the epithelial layer where it is claimed they can help provide support to the skin. Hyaluronic acid is also added to these products to assist in attracting and retaining vital moisture in the form of water in the underlying tissues in order to help keep the collagen and elastin fibres flexible, and also to help plump up the outer layers of the skin.

## Liposomes

Liposomes are minute microspheres which can be suspended within a formula such as a cream. When applied externally, liposomes can be absorbed through the outer dead layers of the skin. Because liposomes have the ability to penetrate right through to the stratum corneum beneath, they can be used to encapsulate a range of active ingredients and deliver them to where they are most required.

## Retin-A (Retinol, Vitamin A)

Retin-A, which is a synthesis of Vitamin A, was initially developed as a treatment for severe cases of acne. Once it became known that this treatment could also result in smoother, younger-looking skin, Retin-A was taken up by the cosmetic industry as the latest miracle solution to ageing skin.

According to dermatologist, Dr David Fenton, of the St John's Centre at St Thomas's Hospital in London, a course of Retin-A treatment can 'permanently eradicate fine wrinkles round the eyes, on the cheeks, and brown marks', and it will have an effect on deeper expression lines. Moreover, Retin-A can help 'generate new blood vessels, stimulate the production of more collagen, normalise damaged epidermal cells, and make the skin rosier, smoother and firmer. And,' adds Dr. Fenton, 'it may even reduce the incidence of skin cancer.' But, and this is a very big but, Retin-A can also have some very unpleasant side-effects such as peeling, dryness, redness, and irritation and can also increase your skin's sensitivity to the sun.

Numerous scientific tests have been applied to Vitamin A and many of its derivatives in order to ascertain and measure how and why it works. There is little doubt today that retinoids in general can prevent connective tissue atrophy, repair skin damage, and even reverse photo-ageing caused by exposure to the sun.

The problem with many over-the-counter preparations

purporting to contain Retin-A is that many simply do not contain enough of the active ingredient to achieve the results that are claimed. And, according to many experts who have examined the bulk of the evidence derived from experiments conducted with stronger-prescription formulas, while Retin-A definitely does effect some improvement, it does not always do so to the extent and with the same degree of consistency that many of its enthusiastic supporters claim.

## Vitamin C

It is now well-established that vitamin C plays a crucial role in the manufacture of collagen within the skin. There is also much anecdotal evidence of its ability to heal wounds, although as little official research has been conducted, this claim has not yet been verified to the satisfaction of scientists.

## Vitamin E

Numerous scientific trials have dispelled many doubts over the need for vitamin E and about its numerous protective and reparative properties when applied topically to the skin. Recent studies indicate that Vitamin E has the capacity to:

- protect and maintain the integrity of the skin's connective tissue
- aid in the prevention of aged skin pigmentation due to free-radical damage
- provide some protection against UV damage
- help repair epidermal damage caused by irradiation
- help prevent loss of water from the skin when applied regularly as a dry-skin moisturiser

One small study was carried out over a four-week period on 20 middle-aged American women using a cream containing a minimum of 5 per cent vitamin E. The results showed a more than a 50-per-cent reduction in the length and depth of crow's feet. Here again, however, the question is: how many products contain sufficient levels of vitamin E to produce results equivalent to those routinely being obtained in trials? Sadly, the answer may well be: far too few.

## Value for Money?

All of the above-mentioned constituents of anti-ageing creams certainly appear to make a surface difference (some quite significantly so) to the appearance and condition of facial skin. It seems, however, that nothing so far discovered has the ability to eliminate all lines, wrinkles, furrows and crow's feet, and in doing so reverse the footprints of time from the surface of our skin.

As to the 64-thousand-dollar question: do these new generation wrinkle-prevention and age-reversal products have anything to offer us? Only a few years ago, women over the age of 30 were not only considered to be over-the-hill, but the effort of climbing the hill was all too evidently etched into their faces. Compare that with the evidence of today, when women of 40, 50, 60, and even beyond are still managing to dazzle with their seemingly youthful complexions, and it is tempting to surmise that the new products are making a real difference. There is, however, another possible explanation.

## A Simple Formula

According to Dr Alexis Carrel who won the Nobel prize for medicine for demonstrating that living cells can be kept alive indefinitely, there is a very simple formula to longevity: 'The cell is immortal. It is merely the fluid in which it floats that degenerates,' he is reported to have said. 'Renew this fluid at intervals, give the cells what they require for nutrition, and as far as we know, the pulsation of life may go on forever.'

Dr Patrick Flanagan, who is Dr Carrel's successor in the field of fluid dynamics, believes that once we uncover the secrets of the special fluid to which Dr Carrel referred, namely cellular water, and find a way to optimise absorption of cellular nutrients, we will have taken a quantum leap in this area of science. Furthermore, while Dr Flanagan, writing in the American journal *Health World*, describes cellular water as being quite different from ordinary water insofar as it is composed of liquid crystals, we nonetheless cannot deny that water – in all its forms – is the matrix of all living things.

And the one thing every cosmetic facial cream has in common, despite all their different formulations of ingredients, is their prime objective is to hydrate the cellular structure of the skin, and to keep any precious moisture they can add to it firmly locked in. In our enthusiasm to pamper our skin by lathering onto its surface literally tons of 'miracle' creams, we may have unwittingly stumbled across the one magical ingredient that really does provide us with the key to rejuvenating our skin. Perhaps we have all been so intent on searching for the 'mythical fountain of youth' that we have somehow failed to see one glaringly obvious clue: it may not be the fountain that is important but the plain and simple substance that every fountain spews forth – namely water. Ultimately, this may prove to provide the solution to the secret of sustaining a strong, healthy body, youthful looks, and an extended life.

# Recommended Reading

Balch, James F. MD and Phyllis A. C.N.C. *Prescription for Nutritional Healing – A Practical A-Z Reference to Drug-Free Remedies Using Vitamins, Minerals, Herbs & Food Supplements* (Avery Publishing Group, USA)

Hendler, Sheldon Saul MD. Ph.D. *The Doctors' Vitamin and Mineral Encyclopedia* (Arrow Books)

Mindell, Earl. *The Vitamin Bible* (Arlington Books)

Free information booklets, leaflets and posters can be obtained by sending a large sae to The Roche Vitamin Information Service, Roche Products Limited, Vitamin & Chemical Division, PO Box 8, Welwyn Garden City, Hertfordshire AL7 3AY

# Index